THE
FAST-FOOD
NUTRITION
·COUNTER·

Annette B. Natow, Ph.D., R.D.
and Jo-Ann Heslin, M.A., R.D.

POCKET BOOKS

New York   London   Toronto   Sydney   Tokyo   Singapore

An *Original* Publication of POCKET BOOKS

POCKET BOOKS, a division of Simon & Schuster Inc.
1230 Avenue of the Americas, New York, NY 10020

Copyright © 1994 by Annette Natow and Jo-Ann Heslin

All rights reserved, including the right to reproduce
this book or portions thereof in any form whatsoever.
For information address Pocket Books, 1230 Avenue
of the Americas, New York, NY 10020

ISBN: 0-671-89475-7

First Pocket Books printing November 1994

10 9 8 7 6 5 4 3 2 1

POCKET and colophon are registered trademarks of
Simon & Schuster Inc.

Cover design by Tom McKeveny

Printed in the U.S.A.

ACKNOWLEDGMENTS

Without the tireless cooperation of Steven and Stephen, *The Fast-Food Nutrition Counter* would never have been completed. Our thanks to the companies and restaurant chains for graciously sharing their information. A special thanks to our editor, Rebecca Todd, and our agent, Nancy Trichter.

"The human being exhibits two psychological tendencies in his diet—one, to stand by the old favorites; the other, to demand variety from day to day."

MARY SWARTZ ROSE, PH.D.
Feeding the Family
The Macmillan Company, 1919

CONTENTS

SOURCES OF DATA

Values in this counter have been obtained from the Composition of Foods, United States Department of Agriculture, Agricultural Handbooks: No. 8-1, Dairy and Egg Products; No. 8-11, Vegetables and Vegetable Products; No. 8-12, Nut and Seed Products; No. 8-14, Beverages; No. 8-18, Baked Products; No. 8-19, Snacks and Sweets; No. 8-21, Fast Foods; Supplements 1989, 1990, 1991, 1992.

Nutritive Value of Foods, United States Department of Agriculture, Home and Garden Bulletin No. 72.

J. Davies and J. Dickerson, *Nutrient Content of Food Portions.* Cambridge, UK: The Royal Society of Chemistry, 1991.

G. A. Leveille, M. E. Zabik, K. J. Morgan, *Nutrients in Foods.* Cambridge, MA: The Nutrition Guild, 1983.

Information from food labels, manufacturers and processors, and restaurants. The values are based on research conducted through 1994. Nutrient values for restaurant menu items and manufacturers' foods may vary from those listed in this book due to reformulation and regional differences.

INTRODUCTION

Americans eat out an average of almost four times a week, spending about 40 percent of their food dollars eating away from home. Now more than ever, fast-food and family restaurants meet the needs of the nineties. Perfectly suited to today's lifestyle, they can be fast (or more relaxed), fun, nutritious, affordable, and can be found just about everywhere.

Catering to every whim, fast-food and family restaurants are great whether you feel like splurging on fattening treats or you'd rather have a salad with low-calorie dressing. There are choices for everyone.

Kids are courted at these restaurants. They offer children's menu selections, toys, and activities. When you are looking for a convenient, enjoyable spot for a children's party, fast-food and family restaurants fit the bill. Besides serving favorite foods, they provide favors like hats and balloons, and often have play areas (sometimes with attendants). Family restaurants provide children with crayons, paper place mats with creative games to keep them busy, and special treats to end the meal. These keep the children happy while the adults enjoy a more relaxed meal.

Teens, especially boys, seem to be hungry all the time. Three meals a day just don't seem to satisfy them. Fast-food and family restaurants are great places for the "fourth meal" of the day that is often needed to fill them up.

Fast-food and family restaurants are also tuned into environmental, social, humanitarian, and health issues. By summer 1994, smoking will be banned in all company-owned Arby's quick-serve restaurants. Other restaurant chains are considering similar action. Food packaging has been changed to reduce waste and recycle more materials, and many franchises actively support local youth activities and athletic teams. Families of critically ill children benefit from the Ronald McDonald houses established by the McDonald Corporation.

Fast-food and family restaurants were among the first to voluntarily offer nutrition information for their menus. Many supply menu selection advice for people who must monitor their diets because of diabetes or high blood pressure. Some even supply special menus for the hearing and vision impaired. Restaurant chains were also among the first to recognize and accommodate multicultural diversity among their customers. They are ready employers of teens, seniors, and others, including those who are developmentally disabled.

FAST FACT
Kids aged 6 to 14 eat in fast-food restaurants 157 million times a month. Those living in the South eat there twice as often as kids in the West.

Singles, young and old, often find it inconvenient to shop for and prepare food for just one person. It's simpler and takes less time to buy a meal already prepared, to take out and eat at home, or to enjoy eating in a restaurant. For the college set, family restaurants offer an affordable opportunity to "dine out" and escape from the campus cafeteria.

Times have changed. Today only 10 percent of households have traditional homemakers who are not employed outside the home. Working adults, with and without children, account for the vast majority of households. They welcome the convenience of having their evening meal prepared for them. Eating at a restaurant, ordering in, or simply picking up all or part of their dinner, already prepared, simplifies their busy lives.

Older folks are catered to at fast-food and family restaurants. There are senior meal selections and senior discounts offered daily and/or on special senior days. Breakfast clubs provide a sociable meal that may sometimes be followed by bingo. Many of these restaurants employ seniors and try to make the environment even more welcoming to older people.

After a morning walk, jog, or workout at the gym, a stop at a fast-food or family restaurant is a pleasant opportunity to refuel and be rewarded for your effort, as we've seen President Clinton do when he wants to press the flesh after jogging.

FAST FACT
In the United States alone there are more than half a million places to eat out.

EATING OUT, EATING WELL

To have a healthy diet, choose a variety of foods, have moderate portions, and balance the foods you eat throughout the day. That's easy to do when you eat in fast-food and family restaurants. A wide selection of foods is available, and new and seasonal foods are often added to the menu. Mexican foods are very popular and many chains now serve them. A bean burrito might be a nice change from your usual hamburger and will add variety as well as fiber to your diet.

Eating moderate portions is really very easy. All foods served in restaurants are portion controlled. A hamburger eaten on Monday will be the same size as one eaten on Thursday. If portion control is an issue for you, staying with a single instead of a double or triple burger is the best choice. If you want more, you'll have to order seconds, a delaying tactic that can keep you from overeating. It's much easier to get more at home.

When you have eaten a high-calorie, high-fat lunch, balance it with lighter foods at other meals during that day or even the next day. If your meal did not have much fruit or vegetables, try to have some later on. It's not hard to eat healthier. Add fruit juice, a steamed vegetable, a baked potato, or a salad with low-fat dressing or a squeeze of lemon.

How About Chicken?

You can usually get grilled or broiled chicken at most restaurants. It's a good idea to remove the skin from the chicken before you eat it. Save fried chicken and chicken nuggets for "once in a blue moon."

On a chicken sandwich, hold the creamy dressing and substitute mustard, salsa, ketchup, or barbecue sauce. Adding lettuce and tomato adds taste, nutrients, and fiber.

How About Pizza?

Choose pizza topped with broccoli, tomatoes, onions, peppers, and mushrooms, reserving pepperoni, sausage, and other meat toppings for once in a while. Hungry enough for two slices? Have one with a vegetable topping along with one other of your choice. Or try just one slice along with a large tossed salad.

FAST FACT
Pizza originated in the early 1700s in Naples, Italy.

How About Hamburgers?

A plain hamburger, topped with lettuce, tomatoes, onions, pickles, ketchup, and/or mustard is the best choice. If you love the larger combo burgers or cheeseburgers, why not share one with a friend and order a large salad or baked potato as a side dish.

How About Fish?

Choose broiled or grilled fish often, saving battered or breaded fried fish for every now and then. Do the same with shrimp; make boiled or steamed (as in cocktails and salads) or broiled shrimp your first choice.

How About Fries?

Fries are a favorite side dish, but try to stick to a small portion. You should also try substituting rice or a baked potato, plain or topped with margarine, chives, and bacon bits.

How About Sandwiches?

Choose multigrain breads and rolls. Go easy on the creamy sauces. Go heavy on lettuce, onion, sprouts, grated carrots, and tomatoes. Try spicy mustard or salsa instead of mayonnaise for a new taste treat.

FAST FACT
Since the 1940s ham and cheese sandwiches have topped the list of favorite sandwiches.

How About Desserts?

Lowfat frozen yogurt with fruit topping is becoming widely available and makes a refreshing and delicious way to end a meal. Some restaurants offer fresh fruit and flavored gelatin at the salad bar. These are great desserts. If you can't resist the double chocolate layer cake, split it or take half home.

How About Breakfast?

The most important thing about breakfast is *eating* it— 40 percent of adults and 25 percent of kids don't. Breakfast is moving out of the home. In 1992, breakfast foods were the fastest-growing segment in food service. This can range from a full sit-down meal to a cup of convenience-store coffee plus a one-handed food item like a roll or muffin, which is estimated to be breakfast for as many as 25 percent of commuters.

You can eat out and have a different breakfast every day. A bagel—easy on the cream cheese; waffles or pancakes— have syrup, skip the sausage; scrambled egg on whole-wheat toast—don't forget cereal with lowfat milk. Add hot chocolate, fruit juice, or a fat-free muffin to any of these.

SNACKING

FAST FACT
According to the Snack Food Association of America, Americans consume 4.75 billion pounds of snack foods a year. An average person eats more than twenty pounds.

Snacking is the great American pastime. It's been estimated that the average American nibbles the equivalent of a fourth meal every day. In fact, because of busy lifestyles, many of us are now snacking on small meals throughout the day, or "grazing," instead of having "three squares." And, no matter what you may have heard, eating as many as six to ten good snacks a day may be healthier. Your body functions best when it doesn't go for long periods without food. Having several small meals helps control appetite and weight, lowers cholesterol levels, improves digestion in older adults, and prevents wide swings in blood sugar levels in people with diabetes.

People of all ages benefit from snacking. Small children, because they fill up so quickly, need between-meal snacks to keep them satisfied. Teenaged boys, because they are growing so fast, require so much food that they benefit from snacks in addition to their meals. Athletes perform better when they have a high-carbohydrate snack before a game or an event. During pregnancy, the increased nutrients needed for the developing baby make snacking smart. Because of body changes, the digestive capacity of older adults may be overwhelmed by large amounts of food. Eating smaller amounts throughout the day is better.

Snacks provide lots of nutrients in addition to calories Yogurt is an excellent source of calcium and other minerals and vitamins; popcorn or nuts add fiber; pretzels and breadsticks have carbohydrates and vitamins; peanut butter has protein; fruits and vegetables—fresh, canned or dried—contain vitamins and fiber. And all snacks offer a pleasant break and boost energy, alertness, and productivity.

The time between eating can be as long as six hours or

more, especially in the afternoon. Studies show that not eating for such a long time decreases productivity on the job and increases accidents. According to researchers, a midafternoon snack is an excellent mental perk. Students who snacked on either candy or yogurt fifteen minutes before exams had better memory and were more alert than students who did not snack. Another study showed that children in the primary grades who snacked on nuts and raisins had better attitudes toward school.

FAST FACT
Shoppers and hotel guests will have more opportunities to eat at their favorite quick-serve restaurants. Major fast-food chains are moving into supermarkets, discount stores, and hotels.

ETHNIC EATING

Part of the fun of eating out is having food that is different from what you eat at home. That's why ethnic eating is so popular. Chinese, Italian, and Mexican are the most popular ethnic-food restaurants. Along with French, Greek, and Indian restaurants, they offer a variety of healthy, tasty choices.

FAST FACT
Dining out is an ancient practice. In Egypt in 512 B.C., a restaurant offered a single dish of wild fowl, cereal, and onions.

Chinese Food

Ask for steamed dumplings instead of deep-fried appetizers, and clear soups instead of egg drop. Choose stir-fried, boiled, or steamed main dishes with a side of plain boiled white or brown rice. When you have fried noodles or wontons, egg rolls, lobster Cantonese, spareribs, duck, or dishes with nuts, split them with others so that you have a smaller portion. If you are watching your salt intake, ask that the food be prepared with no salt or MSG, then season it yourself with light soy sauce, mustard, or duck sauce. Sherbet, pineapple chunks, or lychees with a fortune cookie can be a good way to top off your meal.

Italian Food

Start with a mixed salad, lightly dressed with vinegar and oil, minestrone soup, or a steamed artichoke. Have pasta topped with sautéed or roasted vegetables or with plain tomato sauce (marinara). Other good choices are pasta and beans (pasta e fagioli) and chicken cacciatore. If you sprinkle on grated cheese, use a small amount, just enough for flavor. When you want a creamy topping or a meat or shellfish sauce, split it with others or take half home. Instead of garlic bread, have plain bread or breadsticks. Italian ices, sorbets and fruit poached in wine are good dessert choices.

Mexican/Spanish Food

Start with bean soup or gazpacho and go easy on the nachos. Bean burritos with a little cheese, chicken on soft tacos, and rice and beans are good choices. Lean beef or chicken fajitas with steamed tortillas are fine, but limit the refried beans, sour cream, and guacamole (avocado) toppings. Use salsa, pico de gallo, red sauce, green sauce, or chopped salad to dress the fajitas instead.

French Food

Choose steamed mussels or other shellfish, grilled fresh fish or broiled lean meat. Try chicken with a low-fat sauce like Marengo or Diablo. French bread, without butter, is great for mopping up the sauce. Have a Niçoise salad, a tasty tuna dish. Fresh fruit and a small portion of cheese is a good, traditional dessert.

Greek Food

Lentil soup or grape leaves stuffed with rice are great for starters. Ask for a Greek salad that is light on the feta cheese and heavy on tomatoes. Or have some cucumbers dressed with yogurt. A lamb roast and grilled or roasted chicken are better choices than casseroles of moussaka or pastitsio, which are better shared. Have kabobs of chicken or lamb and vegetables, with rice on the side.

Indian Food

Start with mulligatawny (lentil) soup, a chickpea appetizer, or a mixed-bean salad. Share an order of samosas, fried pastries filled with peas and potatoes. Barbecued chicken or seafood cooked in a tandoor, and chicken or seafood curry are good choices, along with rice and stewed vegetables. Try lentil puree (dal) for a tasty change from meat. Condiments like chutney add flavor and are low in fat. A salad of cucumbers with yogurt is refreshing, as is lassi, a yogurt-based drink. Choose baked and steamed breads instead of fried flatbreads.

FAST FACT
People living in Miami, Washington, D.C., and New York City spend the most on restaurant food.

EATING IN BY TAKING OUT

Take-out food is a major eating trend of the nineties. In 1992, almost half of all restaurant purchases were take-out. Delis, supermarkets, and most restaurants offer a wide selection of take-out foods. This is an easy and economical way of eating dishes that you may not have the skill or time to prepare. When you're short of time, take *in* a main dish and serve it with a salad or fresh fruit. Because take-out foods often do not have nutritional analysis, in Part II, "Take-Out Foods," you'll find a wide selection of items to help you make good choices.

FAST FACT
Eighty percent of all households in the U.S. have microwave ovens, making it simple to heat take-out food. By the year 2001, that number will increase to 95 percent. It's predicted

that soon new cars will come equipped with microwave ovens.

IF YOU HAVE HEALTH CONCERNS

Have you been advised to lose weight, lower your fat intake, or eat less salt? You can eat healthy foods and follow these diet recommendations when you eat in fast-food and family restaurants.

All the foods we eat are combinations of protein, fat, carbohydrates, vitamins, minerals, and fiber. We all need to get enough of these nutrients to stay healthy.

Protein

Don't worry about getting enough protein. Restaurant meals usually have lots of protein in foods like hamburgers, steak, fish, cheese, milk, yogurt, and eggs. Most of us get nearly twice as much as we need. And more is not always better. Too much protein does not make you stronger and may even cause more calcium to be lost from the body, setting the stage for adult bone loss (osteoporosis) later in life.

Fat

While many of us may be eating more fat than is good for us, this doesn't mean that some high-fat food or even one high-fat meal is so bad. It's only part of your overall intake. You can balance it by eating lowfat foods—fruit, vegetables, lowfat milk—at other meals. If, on the other hand, you have been told by your doctor to reduce your fat intake for medical reasons, keep closer tabs on what you eat and avoid very fatty foods whenever you can. This book will help you pick lowfat take-out and restaurant foods so that you can stay within the recommended guideline of no more than 30 percent of your daily calories from fats. Remember that individual foods need not meet this guideline, but overall fat intake for the day should come close. Balance the extra fat in a cheeseburger by choosing a fat-free dressing for your side salad.

Meat, poultry, milk, eggs, cheese, and butter all contain cholesterol. In fact, every food that comes from an animal contains cholesterol. To stay within the recommended intake of 300 milligrams of cholesterol a day, balance your cholesterol-containing menu choice with cholesterol-free food plants—salad, vegetables, margarine, beans, potatoes, pasta, and bread.

Carbohydrates

These are the starches and sugars in your food. We know now that starch does not deserve its bad, fattening reputation. Eating more starch can actually help you lose weight if you don't dress it with lots of fatty add-ons. Pizza, bread, rolls, rice, noodles, and pasta are foods that contain starch and also supply vitamins and minerals.

What about sugar? You really don't have to worry about it unless you have diabetes. In that case discuss sugar with your doctor. While it isn't good to overdo sweets, having a sweet dessert at the end of a meal or as an occasional snack is fun and won't hurt.

When you reduce fat, carbohydrates take up the slack. Aim for 50 percent of your daily calories from carbohydrates. Choose two small burgers, with more carbohydrate from bread, instead of a super burger heavy in meat.

Fiber

Americans eat too little fiber. You can increase your intake by eating more whole grains, fruits, vegetables, beans, and seeds. Eating whole fruits and vegetables instead of drinking their juices is one easy way to boost your fiber intake. Another is to choose whole-grain or multigrain rolls instead of plain rolls.

Vitamins and Minerals

When you eat a variety of different foods, you increase

your chances of getting all the vitamins and minerals you need for good health. Eating more fruits, vegetables, and grains helps. Some foods are better sources of certain vitamins and minerals. For example, milk and yogurt are excellent sources of calcium. But many other foods, like vegetables and nuts, contain this mineral too. Even a food additive commonly added to bread and rolls to keep them fresh contains a little calcium. We all know that orange juice is an excellent source of vitamin C, but you may not know that sliced tomato, green peppers, and baked potatoes are good sources too.

Sodium is a mineral that we often get too much of. Aim for 2400 to 3000 milligrams a day. Don't sprinkle on extra salt, ask for fries minus the salt, choose low-sodium/salt dressing when available, and go easy on sauces. Instead, try a sprinkle of pepper, a squeeze of lemon, or a dash of salsa or hot sauce.

USING YOUR FAST-FOOD NUTRITION COUNTER

FAST FACT
In 1971, there were an estimated 30,000 fast food places in the country, in 1979 there were 140,000.

This book lists the nutrient content of foods served in over 55 restaurant chains, and of 260 take-out foods and over 2500 snacks. For the first time, information about these nutrient values is at your fingertips. Before *The Fast-Food Nutrition Counter* it was impossible to compare so many restaurant and snack foods at one time. For example, when you want to have pizza, you'll find it under the different restaurants that serve it and also among the take-out foods. The choice is up to you.

The Fast-Food Nutrition Counter is divided into three sections. Part I, "Fast-Food and Family Restaurant Chains," lists the nutrient values in restaurant foods. Part II lists nutrient values in "Take-Out Foods" and Part III, "Snacks," gives the nutrient values in eighteen different snack categories. Over 5300 foods are represented in these three lists.

In Part I restaurant chains are listed alphabetically from Arby's through Winchell's. Within each restaurant list, menu items are grouped into categories such as BAKED SELECTIONS, BEVERAGES, BREAKFAST SELECTIONS, CHILDREN'S MENU SELECTIONS, DESSERTS, ICE CREAM, MAIN MENU SELECTIONS, SALAD DRESSINGS, and SALADS AND SALAD BAR.

In Part II take-out food is listed alphabetically in categories from BEANS to VEGETABLES, MIXED. Under BEANS you'll find foods like refried beans and four-bean salad. In the mixed vegetable category there are samosas and ratatouille.

In Part III snacks are listed alphabetically, in categories from BEER AND ALE to YOGURT, FROZEN. This listing gives you nutrient values for most foods that you eat on the run. For each snack category you will find brand-name foods listed first, in alphabetical order, followed by an alphabetical list of generic foods. Miscellaneous and single-listing items, including such diverse snacks as apple chips, Cheetos, Combos, cornnuts, pork skins, and snack mixes, are listed under the general heading MUNCHIES.

Discrepancies in figures are due to rounding. All figures for calories, fat, carbohydrates, cholesterol, and sodium have been rounded to the nearest whole number.

The following pages contain brief definitions of specific terms, abbreviations used throughout this book, and a chart of equivalent measures to help you calculate portions not listed for individual foods.

DEFINITIONS

as prep (as prepared): refers to food that has been prepared according to package directions

take-out: describes prepared dishes that you purchase ready-to-eat; those included serve as a guide to the nutrient values of similar products you may purchase

trace (tr): value used when a food contains less than one calorie, less than one g (gram) of fat or carbohydrate, or less than one mg (milligram) of cholesterol or sodium

ABBREVIATIONS

CAL	=	calories
CARB	=	carbohydrates
CHOL	=	cholesterol
diam	=	diameter
fl oz	=	fluid ounce
frzn	=	frozen
g	=	gram
gal	=	gallon
lb	=	pound
lg	=	large
med	=	medium
mg	=	milligram
oz	=	ounce
pkg	=	package
pt	=	pint
prep	=	prepared
qt	=	quart
reg	=	regular
serv	=	serving
sm	=	small
SOD	=	sodium
sq	=	square
tbsp	=	tablespoon
tr	=	trace
tsp	=	teaspoon
w/	=	with
w/o	=	without
in	=	inch
<	=	less than

EQUIVALENT MEASURES

Dry

3 teaspoons	=	1 tablespoon
4 tablespoons	=	¼ cup
8 tablespoons	=	½ cup
12 tablespoons	=	¾ cup
16 tablespoons	=	1 cup
1000 milligrams	=	1 gram
28 grams	=	1 ounce
4 ounces	=	¼ pound
8 ounces	=	½ pound
12 ounces	=	¾ pound
16 ounces	=	1 pound

Liquid

2 tablespoons	=	1 ounce
2 ounces	=	¼ cup
4 ounces	=	½ cup
6 ounces	=	¾ cup
8 ounces	=	1 cup
2 cups	=	1 pint
2 pints	=	1 quart

THE
FAST-FOOD
NUTRITION
·COUNTER·

PART I

FAST-FOOD AND FAMILY RESTAURANT CHAINS

ALL FAT VALUES ARE GIVEN IN GRAMS (G)
ALL CARBOHYDRATE VALUES ARE GIVEN IN GRAMS
ALL CHOLESTEROL VALUES ARE GIVEN IN MILLIGRAMS (MG)
ALL SODIUM VALUES ARE GIVEN IN MILLIGRAMS
A DASH (—) INDICATES DATA WAS NOT AVAILABLE

FAST FACT
Fast food refers to the service of the food, not the food itself.
It can include any type of food. A more appropriate name
for an establishment serving such foods would be quick-
service restaurant.

FOOD	PORTION	CAL	FAT	CARB	CHOL	SOD

ARBY'S

BAKED SELECTIONS

FOOD	PORTION	CAL	FAT	CARB	CHOL	SOD
Apple Turnover	1	303	18	28	0	178
Blueberry Turnover	1	320	19	32	0	240
Cheesecake	1 serv	306	23	21	95	220
Cherry Turnover	1	280	18	25	0	200
Chocolate Chip Cookie	1	130	4	17	0	95

BEVERAGES

FOOD	PORTION	CAL	FAT	CARB	CHOL	SOD
Chocolate Shake	12 fl oz	451	12	77	36	410
Coca-Cola Classic	12 oz	141	0	38	0	15
Coffee	8 oz	3	0	0	0	3
Diet Coke	12 oz	1	0	0	0	30
Diet 7-Up	12 oz	4	0	0	0	22
Hot Chocolate	8 oz	110	1	0	0	120
Iced Tea	16 oz	6	0	1	0	12
Jamocha Shake	11.5 fl oz	368	11	59	35	262
Milk, 2%	8 oz	121	4	12	18	122
Nehi Orange	12 oz	190	0	47	0	21
Orange Juice	6 oz	82	0	20	0	2
Pepsi-Cola	12 oz	159	0	40	0	10
R.C. Cola	12 oz	173	0	43	0	1
R.C. Diet Rite	12 oz	1	0	tr	0	10
R.C. Root Beer	12 oz	173	0	43	0	16
7-Up	12 oz	144	0	38	0	34
Sugar Substitute	1 pkg (0.8 g)	4	0	0	0	5
Upper Ten	12 oz	169	0	42	0	40
Vanilla Shake	11 fl oz	330	12	46	32	686

BREAKFAST SELECTIONS

FOOD	PORTION	CAL	FAT	CARB	CHOL	SOD
Biscuit, Bacon	1	318	18	36	8	904
Biscuit, Ham	1	323	17	34	21	1169

FOOD	PORTION	CAL	FAT	CARB	CHOL	SOD
Biscuit, Plain	1	280	14	34	0	730
Biscuit, Sausage	1	460	32	35	60	1000
Blueberry Muffin	1	200	6	34	22	269
Cinnamon Nut Danish	1	340	10	59	0	230
Croissant, Bacon/Egg	1	389	26	30	221	582
Croissant, Ham/Cheese	1	345	21	29	90	939
Croissant, Mushroom/Cheese	1	493	38	34	116	935
Croissant, Plain	1	260	16	28	49	300
Croissant, Sausage/Egg	1	519	39	29	271	632
Maple Syrup	1.5 oz	120	tr	29	0	52
Platter, Bacon	1	860	32	49	366	1051
Platter, Egg	1	460	24	45	346	491
Platter, Ham	1	518	26	45	374	1177
Platter, Sausage	1	640	41	46	406	861
Toastix	1 serv	420	25	43	20	440
ICE CREAM Polar Swirl Butterfinger	1	457	18	62	28	318
Polar Swirl Heath	1	543	22	76	39	346
Polar Swirl Oreo	1	482	20	66	35	521
Polar Swirl P'nut Butter Cup	1	517	24	61	34	385
Polar Swirl Snickers	1	511	19	73	33	351
MAIN MENU SELECTIONS Arby's Sauce	0.5 oz	15	tr	3	0	113
Au Jus	4 oz	7	0	1	0	750
Bac N'Cheddar Deluxe Sandwich	1	532	33	35	83	422
Baked Potato, Broccoli 'N Cheddar	1	417	18	55	22	1455

FOOD	PORTION	CAL	FAT	CARB	CHOL	SOD
Baked Potato, Butter/ Margarine & Sour Cream	1	463	25	53	40	203
Baked Potato, Deluxe	1	621	36	59	58	1520
Baked Potato, Mushroom & Cheese	1	515	27	58	47	1445
Baked Potato, Plain	1	240	2	50	0	1333
Beef N'Cheddar Sandwich	1	451	20	43	52	955
Cheddar Fries	1 serv (5 oz)	399	22	46	9	443
Chicken Breast Sandwich	1	489	46	48	45	1019
Chicken Cordon Bleu Sandwich	1	658	37	50	65	1824
Chicken Fajita Pita	1	272	9	33	27	887
Curly Fries	1 serv (3.5 oz)	337	18	43	0	167
Fish Fillet Sandwich	1	537	29	47	79	994
French Dip	1	345	12	34	5	678
French Dip 'N Swiss	1	425	18	36	87	1078
French Fries	1 serv	246	13	30	0	114
Grilled Chicken Barbeque Sandwich	1	378	14	45	44	1059
Grilled Chicken Deluxe Sandwich	1	426	21	39	44	877
Ham 'N Cheese Sandwich	1	330	15	33	45	1350
Horsey Sauce	0.5 oz	55	5	3	1	105
Ketchup	0.5 oz	16	0	4	0	143
Light Ham Deluxe	1	255	6	33	30	1037
Light Roast Beef Deluxe	1	294	10	33	42	826
Light Roast Chicken Deluxe	1	263	6	33	39	620

FOOD	PORTION	CAL	FAT	CARB	CHOL	SOD
Light Roast Turkey Deluxe	1	260	5	33	30	1172
Mayonnaise, Cholesterol Free	0.5 oz	90	10	0	0	75
Mustard	0.5 oz	11	1	1	0	160
Philly Beef N' Swiss Sandwich	1	498	26	37	91	1194
Potato Cakes	1 serv	204	12	20	0	397
Roast Beef Sandwich, Giant	1	530	27	41	78	908
Roast Beef Sandwich, Junior	1	218	11	21	23	345
Roast Beef Sandwich, Regular	1	353	15	32	39	588
Roast Beef Sandwich, Super	1	529	28	46	47	798
Roast Chicken Club	1	513	29	40	75	1423
Roast Chicken Deluxe Sandwich	1	373	20	37	—	913
Roast Chicken Salad	1	184	7	11	36	441
Sub Deluxe	1	482	26	38	45	1530
Turkey Deluxe Sandwich	1	399	20	36	39	1047
SALAD DRESSINGS Blue Cheese	2 oz	295	31	3	50	489
Buttermilk Ranch	2 oz	349	39	2	6	471
Honey French	2 oz	322	27	22	0	486
Italian Light	2 oz	23	1	4	0	1110
Thousand Island	2 oz	298	29	10	24	493
Weight Watchers Creamy French	1 oz	48	3	6	0	170
Weight Watchers Creamy Italian	1 oz	29	3	1	0	280

FOOD	PORTION	CAL	FAT	CARB	CHOL	SOD
SALADS AND SALAD BAR						
Cashew Chicken Salad	1	590	37	23	65	1140
Chef Salad	1	210	11	3	115	720
Croutons	0.5 oz	59	2	9	1	155
Garden Salad	1	149	9	2	74	99
SOUPS						
Beef w/ Vegetables & Barley	8 oz	96	3	14	10	996
Boston Clam Chowder	8 oz	207	11	18	28	1157
Cream of Broccoli	8 oz	180	8	19	—	1133
French Onion	8 oz	67	3	7	0	1248
Lumberjack Mixed Vegetable	8 oz	89	4	13	4	1075
Old-Fashioned Chicken Noodle	8 oz	99	2	15	25	929
Pilgrim's Corn Chowder	5 oz	193	11	18	28	1157
Split Pea w/ Ham	8 oz	200	10	21	30	1029
Tomato Florentine	8 oz	244	2	15	2	910
Wisconsin Cheese	8 oz	287	19	19	31	1129

AU BON PAIN

FOOD	PORTION	CAL	FAT	CARB	CHOL	SOD
BAGELS						
Cinnamon Raisin	1	280	1	58	—	550
Onion	1	270	1	54	—	680
Plain	1	270	1	54	—	680
Sesame	1	270	1	54	—	680
BREADS AND ROLLS						
Alpine Roll	1	220	3	43	0	810
Baguette Loaf	1	810	2	166	0	1830
Braided Roll	1	387	11	64	34	1540
Cheese Loaf	1	1670	29	269	75	4140

FOOD	PORTION	CAL	FAT	CARB	CHOL	SOD
Country Seed Roll	1	220	4	37	0	460
Four-Grain Loaf	1	1420	11	57	tr	3050
French Roll	1	320	tr	65	0	710
Hearth Roll	1	250	2	45	0	510
Hearth Sandwich Roll	1	370	3	69	0	600
Multigrain	2 slices	391	3	77	1	2040
Onion Herb Loaf	1	1430	13	263	0	2390
Parisienne Loaf	1	1490	4	306	0	3380
Petit Pain	1	220	tr	44	0	490
Pita Pocket	1	80	tr	18	—	—
Pumpernickel Roll	1	210	2	42	0	1005
Rye	2 slices	374	4	73	1	2170
Rye Roll	1	230	2	44	0	—
Sandwich Croissant	1	300	14	38	35	240
Three-Seed Raisin Roll	1	250	4	46	0	480
Vegetable Roll	1	230	5	40	0	410
COOKIES						
Chocolate Chip	1	280	15	37	25	70
Chocolate Chunk Pecan	1	290	17	36	10	200
Oatmeal Raisin	1	250	9	41	10	230
Peanut Butter	1	290	15	33	10	250
White Chocolate Chunk Pecan	1	300	17	37	10	200
CROISSANTS						
Almond	1	420	25	41	95	250
Apple	1	250	10	38	25	150
Blueberry Cheese	1	380	20	44	60	280
Chocolate	1	400	24	46	35	220
Chocolate Hazelnut	1	480	28	56	35	220

FOOD	PORTION	CAL	FAT	CARB	CHOL	SOD
Cinnamon Raisin	1	390	13	60	35	240
Coconut Pecan	1	440	23	51	45	290
Ham & Cheese	1	370	20	38	55	280
Plain	1	220	10	29	25	240
Raspberry Cheese	1	400	20	49	60	280
Spinach & Cheese	1	290	16	29	45	310
Strawberry Cheese	1	400	20	49	60	280
Sweet Cheese	1	420	23	45	70	310
Turkey & Cheddar	1	410	22	38	70	680
Turkey & Havarti	1	410	21	38	70	630
MUFFINS						
Blueberry	1	390	11	66	40	410
Bran	1	390	11	73	20	940
Carrot	1	450	22	58	15	610
Corn	1	460	17	71	25	510
Cranberry Walnut	1	350	13	53	15	730
Oat Bran Apple	1	400	10	71	0	590
Pumpkin	1	410	16	63	20	500
Whole Grain	1	440	16	68	30	310
SALAD DRESSINGS						
Balsamic Vinaigrette	1 serv (2.25 oz)	311	33	4	1	420
Champagne Vinaigrette	1 serv (2.25 oz)	251	26	3	2	887
County Blue Cheese	1 serv (2.25 oz)	325	31	10	46	660
Honey & Poppy Seed	1 serv (2.25 oz)	354	35	14	2	199
Italian Low Cal	1 serv (2.25 oz)	68	6	3	5	360
Olive Oil Caesar	1 serv (2.25 oz)	255	16	21	tr	857
Parmesan & Pepper	1 serv (2.25 oz)	235	21	6	19	595
Sesame French	1 serv (2.25 oz)	339	27	22	3	857
Tomato Basil	1 serv (2.25 oz)	66	tr	13	0	359

FOOD	PORTION	CAL	FAT	CARB	CHOL	SOD
SALADS AND SALAD BAR						
Chicken, Cracked Pepper Garden	1	100	2	9	25	360
Chicken, Grilled Garden	1	110	2	9	30	330
Chicken Tarragon Garden	1	310	15	11	70	332
Garden, Large	1	40	tr	8	0	20
Garden, Small	1	20	tr	5	0	10
Shrimp Garden	1	102	2	8	105	193
Tuna Garden	1	350	25	11	40	480
SANDWICHES AND FILLINGS						
Bacon	1 serv	140	12	tr	30	465
Brie	1 serv	300	24	3	85	510
Cheddar Cheese	1 serv	110	9	1	30	150
Chicken, Cracked Pepper	1 serv	120	2	1	50	680
Chicken, Grilled	1 serv	130	4	1	60	610
Chicken Tarragon	1 serv	270	15	3	70	304
Country Ham	1 serv	150	7	3	115	970
Herb Cheese	1 serv	290	29	2	90	390
Provolone Cheese	1 serv	155	13	tr	36	180
Roast Beef	1 serv	180	8	1	60	310
Smoked Turkey	1 serv	100	1	0	35	950
Swiss	1 serv	330	24	3	80	230
Tuna Salad	1 serv	310	24	3	40	450
SOUPS						
Beef Barley	1 bowl	112	3	15	18	901
Beef Barley	1 cup	75	2	10	12	600
Chicken Noodle	1 bowl	119	2	14	26	743
Chicken Noodle	1 cup	79	1	9	17	495
Clam Chowder	1 bowl	433	27	36	90	1027

FOOD	PORTION	CAL	FAT	CARB	CHOL	SOD
Clam Chowder	1 cup	289	18	24	60	687
Cream of Broccoli	1 bowl	302	26	18	54	219
Cream of Broccoli	1 cup	201	17	12	36	146
Garden Vegetarian	1 bowl	44	tr	9	0	92
Garden Vegetarian	1 cup	29	tr	6	0	61
Minestrone	1 bowl	158	2	30	2	398
Minestrone	1 cup	105	1	20	1	265
Split Pea	1 bowl	264	2	45	1	453
Split Pea	1 cup	176	1	30	tr	303
Tomato Florentine	1 bowl	92	2	15	0	221
Tomato Florentine	1 cup	61	1	10	0	147
Vegetarian Chili	1 bowl	208	4	37	0	763
Vegetarian Chili	1 cup	139	3	24	0	508

BASKIN-ROBBINS

FOOD	PORTION	CAL	FAT	CARB	CHOL	SOD
Sugar Cone	1	60	1	11	0	45
Waffle Cone	1	140	2	28	0	5
FROZEN YOGURT						
Cafe Mocha	½ cup (4 fl oz)	70	0	16	0	14
Chocolate, Nonfat	½ cup	110	0	23	0	40
Chocolate Vanilla	½ cup	110	0	22	0	40
Dutch Chocolate Chip Bar	1	260	14	28	7	94
Pralines Vanilla Bar	1	250	14	26	7	76
Strawberry, Low-Fat	½ cup	120	1	24	5	40
Strawberry, Nonfat	½ cup	110	0	24	0	40
Wild Cherry	½ cup	70	0	16	0	15
ICE CREAM						
Almond Butter Crunch Light	½ cup	130	6	16	12	—
Butterfinger	½ cup	170	8	22	15	—

FOOD	PORTION	CAL	FAT	CARB	CHOL	SOD
Butter Pecan	½ cup	160	10	14	25	70
Caramel Banana, Fat Free	½ cup	100	0	23	1	—
Cherry Cordial, Sugar Free	½ cup	100	1	21	3	—
Chewy Baby Ruth	½ cup	190	10	21	25	0
Chilly Burgers, Vanilla	1	240	11	32	29	130
Chocolate	½ cup	150	8	18	20	90
Chocolate Almond	½ cup	170	10	15	20	0
Chocolate Chip	½ cup	150	9	15	25	60
Chocolate Chip, Sugar Free	½ cup	100	2	20	4	—
Chocolate Fudge	½ cup	170	9	21	25	100
Chocolate Mousse Royale	½ cup	180	9	21	20	84
Chocolate Raspberry Truffle	½ cup	180	10	21	25	70
Chocolate Vanilla, Fat Free	½ cup	100	0	21	0	60
Chocolate Wonder, Fat Free	½ cup	120	0	26	1	—
Chunky Banana, Sugar Free	½ cup	80	1	17	3	90
Coconut Caramel Nut Light	½ cup	130	5	19	8	75
Cookies N Cream	½ cup	160	10	16	20	65
Double Raspberry Light	½ cup	120	4	19	9	—
Espresso N Cream Light	½ cup	120	5	15	12	75
French Vanilla	½ cup	170	11	15	55	50
Fudge Brownie	½ cup	180	10	20	20	—
Gold Medal Ribbon	½ cup	150	7	20	20	—

FOOD	PORTION	CAL	FAT	CARB	CHOL	SOD
Jamoca Almond Fudge	½ cup	150	8	17	20	65
Jamoca Swirl, Fat Free	½ cup	100	0	22	2	—
Jamoca Swiss Almond, Sugar Free	½ cup	90	2	19	4	100
Just Peachy, Fat Free	½ cup	100	0	22	2	60
Kahlua N Cream	½ cup	160	8	18	10	6
Mint Chocolate Chip	½ cup	150	9	15	25	50
Peanut Butter Chocolate	½ cup	190	12	16	20	80
Pineapple Cheesecake, Fat Free	½ cup	110	0	25	0	—
Pineapple Coconut, Sugar Free	½ cup	90	1	25	3	70
Pistachio Almond	½ cup	160	10	14	20	45
Praline Dream Light	½ cup	130	6	17	11	85
Pralines N Cream	½ cup	160	8	20	20	100
Reese's Peanut Butter Cup	½ cup	170	10	17	20	—
Rocky Road	½ cup	170	8	22	20	75
Strawberry Royal Light	½ cup	110	3	19	9	120
Strawberry, Sugar Free	½ cup	80	1	17	3	70
Thin Mint Chip, Sugar Free	½ cup	90	2	19	4	90
Tiny Toon Adventures Bar, Mint Chocolate Chip	1	230	15	19	17	35
Tiny Toon Adventures Bar, Vanilla	1	210	14	18	18	35
Tiny Toon Adventures Toonwiches, Chocolate	1	330	14	46	33	105

FOOD	PORTION	CAL	FAT	CARB	CHOL	SOD
Tiny Toon Adventures Toonwiches, Vanilla	1	340	16	15	34	65
Vanilla	½ cup	140	8	14	30	65
Vanilla Fudge Light	½ cup	110	4	18	11	—
Very Berry Strawberry	½ cup	120	6	17	15	55
World Class Chocolate	½ cup	160	8	20	20	80
ICES AND ICE POPS						
Daiquiri Ice	1 scoop	140	0	35	0	15
Rainbow Sherbet	1 scoop	160	2	34	6	85
Strawberry Sorbet	½ cup (4 fl oz)	100	0	20	0	20

BEN & JERRY'S

FOOD	PORTION	CAL	FAT	CARB	CHOL	SOD
FROZEN YOGURT						
Apple Pie	½ cup (4 fl oz)	140	3	28	10	55
Banana Strawberry	½ cup	130	2	27	5	30
Blueberry Cheesecake	½ cup	130	2	26	10	40
Cherry Garcia	½ cup	150	3	28	10	40
Chocolate	½ cup	140	3	26	5	40
Chocolate Fudge Brownie	½ cup	170	4	31	10	95
Chocolate Pop	1 (2.5 fl oz)	150	9	17	0	75
Coffee Almond Fudge	½ cup	180	7	28	10	60
Heath Bar Crunch	½ cup	170	6	29	10	80
Raspberry	½ cup	120	2	24	5	35
ICE CREAM						
Cherry Garcia	½ cup (4 fl oz)	230	16	23	80	35
Chocolate	½ cup	230	14	24	55	25
Chocolate Chip Cookie Dough	½ cup	260	17	29	85	65
Chocolate Fudge Brownie	½ cup	250	14	29	50	85

FOOD	PORTION	CAL	FAT	CARB	CHOL	SOD
Chocolate Peanut Butter Chocolate Chip Cookie Dough	½ cup	280	18	28	55	60
Chunky Monkey	½ cup	270	19	27	70	25
Coffee Heath Bar Crunch	½ cup	270	19	26	80	100
Heath Bar Crunch	½ cup	270	19	26	85	100
Mint Cookie	½ cup	250	17	25	85	100
New York Super Fudge	½ cup	290	20	26	45	40
Pop						
Cherry Garcia	1 (3.7 fl oz)	250	18	25	45	100
Chocolate Chip Cookie Dough	1 (2.5 fl oz)	240	16	26	45	110
Heath Bar Crunch	1 (2.5 fl oz)	260	18	25	35	65
Heath Bar Crunch	1 (3.7 fl oz)	340	23	35	50	90
Milk Chocolate Almond	1 (2.5 fl oz)	250	19	16	35	85
New York Super Fudge	1 (3.7 fl oz)	330	26	22	25	135
Rain Forest Crunch	1 (3.7 fl oz)	350	27	26	50	195
Rain Forest Crunch	½ cup	270	21	21	85	100
Vanilla	½ cup	215	16	18	95	30
Vanilla Brownie Bar	1 (4 fl oz)	260	14	32	50	165
Vanilla Chocolate Chunk	½ cup	250	18	24	85	30

BIG BOY

DESSERTS

FOOD	PORTION	CAL	FAT	CARB	CHOL	SOD
Frozen Yogurt	1 serv	72	0	16	0	31
Frozen Yogurt Shake	1 serv	184	tr	36	2	127
No-No Frozen Dessert	1 serv	75	0	17	0	36

FOOD	PORTION	CAL	FAT	CARB	CHOL	SOD
MAIN MENU SELECTIONS						
Baked Cod Dijon Dinner	1 serv	455	19	21	76	585
Baked Cod Dinner	1 serv	392	13	20	76	389
Baked Potato	1	163	tr	37	0	7
Bran Muffin	1	367	10	61	0	604
Breast of Chicken Dinner	1 serv	358	13	20	68	346
Breast of Chicken w/ Mozzarella Dinner	1 serv	379	12	24	79	357
Breast of Chicken w/ Mozzarella Sandwich	1	390	13	26	71	416
Broiled Cod Dijon Dinner	1 serv	455	19	21	76	585
Broiled Cod Dinner	1 serv	392	13	20	76	389
Cajun Chicken Dinner	1 serv	358	13	20	68	616
Cajun Cod Dinner	1 serv	392	13	20	76	479
Carrots	1 serv	35	tr	8	0	38
Chicken Breast Salad w/ Dijon & Pita Bread	1 serv	377	11	31	60	410
Corn	1 serv	90	1	21	0	1
Dijon Sauce	1 serv	63	6	1	0	196
Dinner Salad	1	19	tr	4	0	11
Green Beans	1 serv	28	tr	6	0	1
Mixed Vegetables	1 serv	27	tr	5	0	42
Peas	1 serv	77	tr	13	0	131
Promise Margarine	1 pat (5 g)	35	4	0	0	35
Rice	1 serv	114	tr	25	0	633
Roll	1	139	tr	30	2	187
Spaghetti Marinara Dinner	1 serv	450	6	87	8	761
Stir-Fry Chicken 'n Vegetable Dinner	1 serv	562	14	68	68	750

FOOD	PORTION	CAL	FAT	CARB	CHOL	SOD
Stir-Fry Vegetable	1 serv	408	10	74	0	703
Turkey Pita	1	224	5	24	75	833
Vegetable Pita	1	144	3	25	10	246
SALAD DRESSING Buttermilk	1 serv	36	2	4	10	151
SOUP Cabbage	1 bowl	43	1	9	1	727
Cabbage	1 cup	37	tr	8	1	623

BURGER KING

FOOD	PORTION	CAL	FAT	CARB	CHOL	SOD
BEVERAGES Coca-Cola Classic	1 med (22 fl oz)	264	0	70	0	—
Coffee, Black	1 (8.6 fl oz)	2	0	0	0	2
Diet Coke	1 med (22 fl oz)	1	0	0	0	—
Milk, 2%	1 (8.6 fl oz)	121	5	12	18	122
Orange Juice	1 (6.4 fl oz)	82	0	20	0	2
Shake, Chocolate	1 med (10 fl oz)	320	7	54	20	230
Shake, Chocolate Syrup Added	1 med (11 fl oz)	400	9	68	20	350
Shake, Strawberry Syrup Added	1 med (10.9 fl oz)	370	6	67	20	240
Shake, Vanilla	1 med (10 fl oz)	310	6	53	20	230
Sprite	1 med (22 fl oz)	264	0	66	0	—
BREAKFAST SELECTIONS A.M. Express Dip	1 oz	84	0	21	0	18
Breakfast Buddy w/ Sausage, Egg & Cheese	1 (2.9 oz)	255	16	15	127	492
Cream Cheese	1 serv (1 oz)	98	7	1	25	86
Croissan'wich Bacon, Egg & Cheese	1 (4.1 oz)	353	23	19	230	780
Ham, Egg & Cheese	1 (5.1 oz)	351	22	20	236	1373

FOOD	PORTION	CAL	FAT	CARB	CHOL	SOD
Croissan'wich *(cont.)*						
Sausage, Egg & Cheese	1 (5.6 oz)	534	40	22	258	985
French Toast Sticks	1 serv (4.9 oz)	440	27	60	0	490
Hash Browns	1 serv (2.5 oz)	213	12	25	0	318
Mini Muffins, Blueberry	1 serv (3.3 oz)	292	14	37	72	244
DESSERTS						
Dutch Apple Pie	1 serv (4 oz)	308	15	39	0	228
Popcorn	1 serv (1 oz)	130	6	17	15	540
Snickers Ice Cream Bar	1 (2 oz)	220	14	20	15	65
MAIN MENU SELECTIONS						
American Cheese	1 slice (1 oz)	92	7	1	25	312
Bacon Bits	½ tsp	16	1	0	5	—
Bacon Double Cheeseburger	1 (5.2 oz)	470	28	26	100	800
Bacon Double Cheeseburger Deluxe	1 (6.5 oz)	570	38	26	110	990
Baked Potato	1 (7 oz)	210	0	48	0	15
BK Big Fish Sandwich	1 (8.9 oz)	710	43	58	60	1110
BK Broiler	1 (5.4 oz)	280	10	29	50	770
BK Broiler Sauce	1 serv (0.4 fl oz)	37	4	1	5	74
Bull's Eye Barbecue Sauce	0.5 fl oz	22	0	5	0	47
Butterfly Shrimp	1 serv (4.1 oz)	300	17	21	105	610
Cheeseburger	1 (4 oz)	300	14	28	45	660
Chicken Sandwich	1 (8 oz)	700	42	54	60	1440
Chicken Tenders	6 pieces (3.2 oz)	236	13	14	38	541
Cocktail Sauce	1 serv (0.7 oz)	20	0	4	0	260
Croutons	1 serv (0.2 oz)	31	1	5	46	90
Dinner Roll	1 (0.9 oz)	80	2	13	0	140

FOOD	PORTION	CAL	FAT	CARB	CHOL	SOD
Dipping Sauce						
Barbecue	1 oz	36	0	9	0	397
Honey	1 oz	91	0	23	0	12
Ranch	1 oz	171	18	2	0	208
Sweet & Sour	1 oz	45	0	11	00	52
Double Cheeseburger	1 (5.6 oz)	450	25	29	90	840
Double Whopper	1 (12.3 oz)	860	55	44	170	950
Double Whopper w/ Cheese	1 (13.2 oz)	950	63	16	195	1260
French Fries, Salted	1 med serv (4.1 oz)	372	20	43	0	238
Hamburger	1 (3.6 oz)	260	10	28	30	500
Ketchup	0.5 fl oz	17	0	4	0	183
Lettuce	1 leaf (0.7 oz)	3	0	4	0	2
Mayonnaise	1 oz	210	23	1	20	160
Mustard	½ tsp	2	0	4	0	34
Onion	0.5 oz	5	0	1	0	0
Onion Rings	1 serv (3.4 oz)	339	19	38	0	628
Pickles	0.5 oz	1	0	0	0	119
Sour Cream	1 oz	60	6	1	15	15
Tartar Sauce	1 oz	175	19	0	15	220
Tomato	1 oz	6	0	1	0	3
Whipped Classic Blend	1 serv (0.4 oz)	65	7	0	0	74
Whopper	1 (9.5 oz)	630	38	44	90	880
Whopper Jr.	1 (4.6 oz)	330	19	28	40	500
Whopper Jr. w/ Cheese	1 (5.1 oz)	380	22	29	50	660
Whopper w/ Cheese	1 (10.3 oz)	720	46	46	115	1190
SALAD DRESSINGS						
Bleu Cheese	1 serv (1.1 oz)	150	16	1	29	256
French	1 serv (1.1 oz)	145	11	1	0	200

FOOD	PORTION	CAL	FAT	CARB	CHOL	SOD
Italian Reduced Calorie Light	1 serv (1.1 oz)	15	1	3	0	355
Ranch	1 serv (1.1 oz)	175	18	2	10	158
Thousand Island	1 serv (1.1 oz)	145	13	8	18	202
SALADS AND SALAD BAR						
Chef Salad w/o Dressing	1 (9.6 oz)	178	9	7	103	568
Chunky Chicken Salad w/o Dressing	1 (9.1 oz)	142	4	8	49	443
Dinner Side Salad	1 (3.5 oz)	20	0	4	0	10
Garden Salad w/o Dressing	1 (7.8 oz)	95	5	8	15	125

CAPTAIN D'S

FOOD	PORTION	CAL	FAT	CARB	CHOL	SOD
DESSERTS						
Carrot Cake	1 piece (4 oz)	434	23	49	32	414
Cheesecake	1 piece (4 oz)	420	31	30	141	480
Chocolate Cake	1 piece (4 oz)	303	10	49	20	259
Lemon Pie	1 piece (4 oz)	351	10	59	45	135
Pecan Pie	1 piece (4 oz)	458	20	64	4	373
MAIN MENU SELECTIONS						
Baked Fish Dinner w/ Slaw	1 dinner	451	19	62	105	1767
Baked Potato	1 (9 oz)	277	tr	64	0	20
Breadstick	1 (1.3 oz)	91	1	17	0	210
Breadsticks	6 (7.5 oz)	545	7	102	0	1260
Broiled Chicken Sandwich	1 (8.2 oz)	451	19	29	105	858
Cheese	1 slice (0.5 oz)	54	5	tr	14	206
Chicken Dinner w/ Salad	1 dinner	414	8	55	71	2615
Cob Corn	1 serv (9.5 oz)	251	2	60	0	13
Cocktail Sauce	1 lg serv (4 oz)	137	tr	34	0	1007

FOOD	PORTION	CAL	FAT	CARB	CHOL	SOD
Coleslaw	1 pt (16 oz)	633	47	47	66	454
Coleslaw	1 serv (4 oz)	158	12	12	16	246
Crackers	4	50	1	8	3	147
Cracklins	1 serv (1 oz)	218	17	16	0	741
Creamer	1 serv (0.4 oz)	14	1	1	0	8
Dinner Salad w/o Dressing	1 (2.5 oz)	27	1	3	1	67
French Fried Potatoes	1 serv (3.5 oz)	302	10	50	0	152
Fried Okra	1 serv (4 oz)	300	16	34	0	445
Green Beans, Seasoned	1 serv (4 oz)	46	2	5	4	752
Hushpuppies	6 (6.7 oz)	756	25	119	0	2790
Hushpuppy	1 (1.1 oz)	126	4	20	0	465
Orange Roughy Dinner w/ Salad	1 dinner	537	19	56	39	2156
Rice	1 serv (4 oz)	124	0	28	0	9
Shrimp Dinner w/ Salad	1 dinner	457	10	56	191	2194
Stuffed Crab	1 serv	91	7	16	—	250
Sugar	1 pkg	18	0	3	0	0
Sweet & Sour Sauce	1 lg serv (4 oz)	206	0	52	0	18
Sweet & Sour Sauce	1 serv (1 oz)	52	0	13	0	5
Tartar Sauce	1 lg serv (4 oz)	298	27	13	41	633
Tartar Sauce	1 serv (1 oz)	75	7	3	10	158
White Beans	1 serv (4 oz)	126	1	22	2	99
SALAD DRESSINGS						
Blue Cheese	1 pkg (1 oz)	105	12	tr	14	101
French	1 pkg (1 oz)	111	11	4	7	187
Italian Lo Cal	1 pkg (1 oz)	9	0	tr	0	568
Ranch	1 pkg (1 oz)	92	10	tr	15	230

FOOD	PORTION	CAL	FAT	CARB	CHOL	SOD

CARL'S JR.

BAKED SELECTIONS

FOOD	PORTION	CAL	FAT	CARB	CHOL	SOD
Blueberry Muffin	1 (4.2 oz)	340	9	61	45	300
Bran Muffin	1 (4.7 oz)	310	6	52	60	370
Cheesecake	1 serv (3.5 oz)	310	17	32	60	200
Cheese Danish	1 (4 oz)	520	22	75	0	230
Chocolate Cake	1 serv (3 oz)	300	11	49	25	262
Chocolate Chip Cookie	1 (2.5 oz)	330	17	41	5	170
Cinnamon Roll	1 (4 oz)	460	18	70	0	230
Fudge Moussecake	1 slice (4 oz)	400	23	42	110	85

BEVERAGES

FOOD	PORTION	CAL	FAT	CARB	CHOL	SOD
Iced Tea	1 reg (21 fl oz)	2	0	0	0	0
Milk, 1%	1 (11 fl oz)	150	3	19	13	200
Orange Juice	1 sm (3.2 fl oz)	90	tr	21	0	2
Shake	1 reg (11.6 fl oz)	350	7	61	15	230
Soda	1 reg (21 fl oz)	240	0	62	0	35
Soda, Diet	1 reg (21 fl oz)	2	0	0	0	15

BREAKFAST SELECTIONS

FOOD	PORTION	CAL	FAT	CARB	CHOL	SOD
Bacon	2 strips (0.3 oz)	45	4	0	5	150
Breakfast Burrito	1 (5.3 oz)	430	26	29	285	740
English Muffin w/ Margarine	1 (2.2 oz)	190	5	30	0	280
French Toast Dips w/o Syrup	1 serv (5.4 oz)	450	20	59	40	570
Hash Brown Nuggets	1 serv (3.3 oz)	270	17	27	5	410
Hotcakes w/ Margarine w/o Syrup	1 serv (6.6 oz)	510	24	61	10	950
Sausage	1 patty (1.6 oz)	190	18	0	30	520
Scrambled Eggs	1 serv (2.4 oz)	120	9	2	245	105
Sunrise Sandwich	1 (4.1 oz)	300	13	31	160	550

FOOD	PORTION	CAL	FAT	CARB	CHOL	SOD
MAIN MENU SELECTIONS						
American Cheese	1 serv (0.6 oz)	60	5	1	15	290
Carl's Catch Fish Sandwich	1 (7.4 oz)	560	30	54	5	1220
Carl's Original Hamburger	1 (6.8 oz)	460	20	46	50	810
Charbroiled BBQ Chicken Sandwich	1 (6.7 oz)	310	6	34	30	680
Charbroiled Chicken Club Sandwich	1 (8.8 oz)	570	29	42	60	1160
Chicken Strips	6 pieces (3.7 oz)	260	19	19	25	600
CrissCut Fries	1 reg serv (3.2 oz)	330	22	27	—	890
Double Western Bacon Cheeseburger	1 (11.5 oz)	1030	63	58	145	1810
Famous Star Hamburger	1 (8.6 oz)	610	38	42	50	890
French Fries	1 reg serv (4.4 oz)	420	20	54	0	200
Great Stuffs Potato						
Bacon & Cheese	1 (14.9 oz)	730	43	60	45	1670
Broccoli & Cheese	1 (15 oz)	590	31	60	25	830
Cheese	1 (14.6 oz)	690	36	70	40	1160
Chili	1 (14.3 oz)	500	26	50	50	630
Lite	1 (10 oz)	290	1	60	0	60
Sour Cream & Chives	1 (12.3 oz)	470	19	64	20	180
Hamburger	1 (4.2 oz)	320	14	33	35	590
Onion Rings	1 serv (5.3 oz)	520	26	63	0	960
Roast Beef Deluxe Sandwich	1 (9.3 oz)	540	26	46	40	1340
Salsa	1 oz	8	0	2	0	210
Sante Fe Chicken Sandwich	1 (7.9 oz)	530	29	36	85	500

FOOD	PORTION	CAL	FAT	CARB	CHOL	SOD
Super Star Hamburger	1 (11.2 oz)	820	53	41	105	1210
Swiss Cheese	1 serv (0.6 oz)	60	4	1	15	220
Turkey Club Sandwich	1 (9.3 oz)	530	23	50	60	2890
Western Bacon Cheeseburger	1 (8.1 oz)	730	39	59	90	1490
Zucchini	1 serv (5.9 oz)	390	23	38	0	1040
SALAD DRESSINGS Blue Cheese	1 oz	150	15	0	20	250
French Reduced Calorie	1 oz	40	2	5	0	290
House	1 oz	110	11	2	10	170
Italian Reduced Calorie	1 oz	40	2	5	0	290
Thousand Island	1 oz	110	11	4	5	200
SALADS AND SALAD BAR Chicken Salad-To-Go	1 (12 oz)	200	8	8	70	300
Garden Salad-To-Go	1 (4.8 oz)	50	3	4	5	75

CARVEL

FOOD	PORTION	CAL	FAT	CARB	CHOL	SOD
FROZEN YOGURT Low Fat	4 fl oz	110	2	22	—	90
Lo-Yo	4 fl oz	140	4	22	—	90
ICE CREAM Carvella	4 fl oz	180	10	19	—	100
Chocolate	4 fl oz	180	10	21	—	100
Thinny-Thin	4 fl oz	90	1	18	—	82

CHICK-FIL-A

FOOD	PORTION	CAL	FAT	CARB	CHOL	SOD
BEVERAGES Iced Tea, Unsweetened	1 reg (9 fl oz)	3	tr	0	0	0
Lemonade	1 sm (10 fl oz)	138	tr	32	tr	tr
Lemonade, Diet	1 sm (10 fl oz)	32	tr	8	0	tr

FOOD	PORTION	CAL	FAT	CARB	CHOL	SOD
DESSERTS						
Cheesecake	1 slice (3.2 oz)	299	19	25	13	272
Cheesecake w/ Blueberry Topping	1 slice (4.3 oz)	350	19	37	13	294
Cheesecake w/ Strawberry Topping	1 slice (4.3 oz)	343	19	35	13	309
Fudge Brownie w/ Nuts	1 (2.78 oz)	369	19	45	31	213
Icedream	1 sm (4.5 oz)	134	5	19	24	51
Lemon Pie	1 slice (4.1 oz)	329	5	64	7	300
MAIN MENU SELECTIONS						
Carrot & Raisin Salad	1 serv (2.67 oz)	116	5	18	6	8
Chargrilled Chicken Deluxe Sandwich	1 (7.15 oz)	266	5	26	40	1125
Chargrilled Chicken Garden Salad	1 serv (10.4 oz)	126	2	8	28	567
Chargrilled Chicken Sandwich	1 (5.46 oz)	258	5	24	40	1121
Chargrilled Chicken w/o Bun	1 piece (3.6 oz)	128	2	1	32	698
Chicken Deluxe Sandwich	1 (7.45 oz)	368	9	30	66	1178
Chicken Salad Plate	1 serv (12.6 oz)	291	19	10	7	584
Chicken Salad Sandwich on Whole Wheat	1 (5.7 oz)	365	18	26	8	840
Chicken Sandwich	1 (5.76 oz)	360	9	28	66	1178
Chicken w/o Bun	1 piece (3.6 oz)	219	7	2	42	801
Chick-N-Q Sandwich	1 (6.8 oz)	409	15	41	10	1197
Coleslaw	1 serv (3.72 oz)	175	14	11	13	158
Grilled 'n Lites	2 skewers (2.7 oz)	97	2	tr	3	280
Hearty Breast of Chicken Soup	1 cup (8.5 fl oz)	152	3	11	46	530

FOOD	PORTION	CAL	FAT	CARB	CHOL	SOD
Nuggets	8 pack (4 oz)	287	15	13	61	1326
Potato Salad	1 serv (3.84 oz)	198	15	14	6	337
Waffle Potato Fries	1 sm serv (3 oz)	270	14	33	8	45
SALADS AND SALAD BAR						
Tossed Salad	1 serv (4.5 oz)	21	tr	4	0	19
Tossed Salad w/ Blue Cheese Dressing	1 serv (6 oz)	243	24	6	38	475
Tossed Salad w/ Honey French Dressing	1 serv (6 oz)	277	21	21	0	396
Tossed Salad w/ Italian Lite Dressing	1 serv (6 oz)	43	1	7	0	856
Tossed Salad w/ Ranch Dressing	1 serv (6 oz)	298	30	6	5	387
Tossed Salad w/ Ranch Lite Dressing	1 serv (6 oz)	114	6	13	6	292
Tossed Salad w/ Thousand Island Dressing	1 serv (6 oz)	250	22	12	25	396

CHURCH'S FRIED CHICKEN

FOOD	PORTION	CAL	FAT	CARB	CHOL	SOD
Apple Pie	1 serv (3.1 oz)	280	12	41	<5	340
Biscuit	1 serv (2.1 oz)	250	16	26	<5	640
Breast	1 serv (2.8 oz)	200	12	4	65	510
Cajun Rice	1 serv (3.1 oz)	130	7	15	5	260
Coleslaw	1 serv (3 oz)	92	6	8	0	230
Corn on the Cob	1 serv (5.7 oz)	190	5	32	0	15
French Fries	1 serv (2.7 oz)	210	11	29	0	60
Leg	1 serv (2 oz)	140	9	3	45	160
Okra	1 serv (2.8 oz)	210	16	19	0	520
Potatoes & Gravy	1 serv (3.7 oz)	90	3	14	0	520
Thigh	1 serv (2.8 oz)	230	16	5	80	520
Wing	1 serv (3.1 oz)	250	16	8	60	540

FOOD	PORTION	CAL	FAT	CARB	CHOL	SOD

DAIRY QUEEN / BRAZIER

FOOD SELECTION

FOOD	PORTION	CAL	FAT	CARB	CHOL	SOD
BBQ Beef Sandwich	1	225	4	34	20	700
Breaded Chicken Fillet Sandwich	1	430	20	37	55	760
Breaded Chicken Fillet Sandwich w/ Cheese	1	480	25	38	70	980
Double Hamburger	1	460	25	29	95	630
Double Hamburger w/ Cheese	1	570	34	31	120	1070
DQ Homestyle Ultimate Burger	1	700	47	30	140	1110
Fish Fillet Sandwich	1	370	16	39	45	630
Fish Fillet Sandwich w/ Cheese	1	420	21	40	60	850
French Reduced Calorie Dressing	2 oz	90	5	11	0	450
French Fries	1 lg serv	390	18	52	0	200
French Fries	1 reg serv	300	14	40	0	160
French Fries	1 sm serv	210	10	29	0	115
Garden Salad w/o dressing	1	200	13	7	185	240
Grilled Chicken Fillet Sandwich	1	300	8	33	50	800
Hot Dog	1	280	16	23	25	700
Hot Dog w/ Cheese	1	330	21	24	35	920
Hot Dog w/ Chili	1	320	19	26	30	720
Lettuce	0.5 oz	2	0	0	0	1
Onion Rings	1 reg	240	12	29	0	135
Quarter-Pound Hot Dog	1	590	38	41	60	1360
Side Salad w/o dressing	1	25	0	4	0	15

FOOD	PORTION	CAL	FAT	CARB	CHOL	SOD
Single Hamburger	1	310	13	29	45	580
Single Hamburger w/ Cheese	1	365	18	30	60	800
Thousand Island Dressing	2 oz	225	21	10	25	570
Tomato	0.5 oz	3	0	1	0	1
ICE CREAM Banana Split	1	510	11	93	30	250
Blizzard, Strawberry	1 reg	740	16	92	50	230
Blizzard, Strawberry	1 sm	500	12	64	35	160
Breeze, Strawberry	1 reg	590	1	90	5	170
Breeze, Strawberry	1 sm	400	tr	63	5	115
Buster Bar	1	450	29	40	15	220
Cone, Chocolate	1 lg	350	11	54	30	170
Cone, Chocolate	1 reg	230	7	36	20	115
Cone, Dipped Chocolate	1 reg	330	16	40	20	100
Cone, Vanilla	1 lg	340	10	53	30	140
Cone, Vanilla	1 reg	230	7	36	20	95
Cone, Vanilla	1 sm	140	4	22	15	60
Cone, Yogurt	1 lg	260	tr	56	5	115
Cone, Yogurt	1 reg	180	tr	38	<5	80
Cup, Yogurt	1 lg	230	tr	49	<5	100
Cup, Yogurt	1 reg	170	tr	35	<5	70
Dilly Bar	1	210	13	21	10	50
DQ Frozen Cake Slice, Undecorated	1	380	18	50	20	210
DQ Sandwich	1	140	4	24	5	135
Heath Blizzard	1 reg	820	36	114	60	410
Heath Blizzard	1 sm	560	23	79	40	280
Heath Breeze	1 reg	680	21	113	15	360

FOOD	PORTION	CAL	FAT	CARB	CHOL	SOD
Heath Breeze	1 sm	450	12	78	10	230
Hot Fudge Brownie Delight	1	710	29	102	35	340
Malt, Vanilla	1 reg	610	14	106	45	230
Mr. Misty	1 reg	250	0	63	0	0
Nutty Double Fudge	1	580	22	85	35	170
Peanut Buster Parfait	1	710	32	94	30	410
QC Big Scoop, Chocolate	1	310	14	40	35	100
QC Big Scoop, Vanilla	1	300	14	39	35	100
Shake, Chocolate	1 reg	540	14	94	45	290
Shake, Vanilla	1 lg	600	16	101	50	260
Shake, Vanilla	1 reg	520	14	88	45	230
Sundae, Chocolate	1 reg	300	7	54	20	140
Sundae, Strawberry Yogurt	1 reg	200	tr	43	<5	80
Sundae, Strawberry Waffle Cone	1	350	12	56	20	220

D'ANGELO SANDWICH SHOPS

FOOD	PORTION	CAL	FAT	CARB	CHOL	SOD
ICE CREAM						
Banana Frozen Yogurt	5 oz	125	3	—	32	60
Banana Frozen Yogurt w/ Cone	5 oz	215	4	—	32	60
Peach Frozen Yogurt	5 oz	130	3	—	31	55
Peach Frozen Yogurt w/ Cone	5 oz	220	3	—	31	60
SALADS AND SALAD BAR						
Beef	1 serv	350	5	—	63	890
Chicken	1 serv	325	4	—	49	980
Tuna	1 serv	305	2	—	32	805
Turkey	1 serv	375	4	—	64	660

FOOD	PORTION	CAL	FAT	CARB	CHOL	SOD
SANDWICHES AND FILLINGS						
D'Lite Pocket						
Chicken Stir Fry	1	340	4	—	60	1025
Roast Beef	1	325	5	—	63	730
Steak	1	415	11	—	91	500
Steak & Mushroom	1	420	11	—	91	620
Steak & Peppers	1	420	11	—	91	500
Turkey	1	350	4	—	64	500
Vegetarian	1	350	11	—	26	995
D'Lite Small Sub						
Roast Beef	1	365	7	—	63	750
DEL TACO						
BEVERAGES						
Coca-Cola Classic	1 lg	287	0	76	0	35
Coca-Cola Classic	1 med	198	0	52	0	24
Coca-Cola Classic	1 sm	144	0	38	0	17
Coca-Cola Classic Best Value	1 serv	395	0	104	0	48
Coffee	1 serv	6	tr	1	0	4
Diet Coke	1 lg	2	0	tr	0	39
Diet Coke	1 med	1	0	tr	0	27
Diet Coke	1 sm	1	0	tr	0	20
Diet Coke Best Value	1 serv	2	0	tr	0	53
Iced Tea	1 lg	6	tr	2	0	26
Iced Tea	1 med	4	tr	1	0	18
Iced Tea	1 sm	3	tr	tr	0	13
Iced Tea Best Value	1 serv	8	tr	2	0	36
Milk	1	126	3	15	12	152
Mr. Pibb	1 lg	283	0	72	0	47
Mr. Pibb	1 med	195	0	49	0	32
Mr. Pibb	1 sm	142	0	36	0	23

FOOD	PORTION	CAL	FAT	CARB	CHOL	SOD
Mr. Pibb Best Value	1 serv	390	0	99	0	64
Orange Juice	1	83	tr	2	0	19
Shake Chocolate	1 med	755	22	135	55	415
Shake, Chocolate	1 sm	549	16	98	40	302
Shake, Orange	1 med	837	22	162	55	322
Shake, Orange	1 sm	609	16	118	40	234
Shake, Strawberry	1 med	668	22	120	55	305
Shake, Strawberry	1 sm	486	16	87	40	222
Shake, Vanilla	1 med	707	25	121	63	353
Shake, Vanilla	1 sm	514	18	88	46	257
Sprite	1 lg	287	0	72	0	71
Sprite	1 med	198	0	49	0	49
Sprite	1 sm	144	0	36	0	35
Sprite Best Value	1 serv	395	0	99	0	97
BREAKFAST SELECTIONS						
Burrito, Beef & Egg	1	529	27	43	328	929
Burrito, Breakfast	1	256	11	30	90	409
Burrito, Egg & Bean	1	470	22	45	305	1035
Burrito, Egg & Cheese	1	443	22	40	305	792
Burrito, Steak & Egg	1	500	25	41	337	1068
CHILDREN'S MENU SELECTIONS						
Kid's Meal Hamburger	1	617	20	97	29	799
Kid's Meal Taco	1	532	17	87	16	373
ICE CREAM						
M&Ms Toppers	1	256	8	42	19	112
Oreos Toppers	1	257	10	42	19	188
Snickers Toppers	1	254	10	41	18	128
MAIN MENU SELECTIONS						
American Cheese	1 slice	53	4	tr	14	203
Beans & Cheese	1	122	3	17	9	892

FOOD	PORTION	CAL	FAT	CARB	CHOL	SOD
Burrito						
Chicken	1	264	10	32	36	771
Combination	1	413	17	46	49	1035
Del Beef	1	440	20	43	63	878
Deluxe Chicken	1	549	34	40	83	978
Deluxe Combo	1	453	20	49	59	1047
Deluxe Del Beef	1	479	23	45	73	890
Green	1	229	8	32	15	714
Green, Regular	1	330	11	46	22	1149
Macho Beef	1	893	41	84	139	1969
Macho Combo	1	774	31	87	100	2180
Red	1	235	8	32	17	656
Red, Regular	1	324	12	46	26	1033
Cheeseburger	1	284	13	26	42	852
Chicken Salad	1	254	19	8	58	476
Chicken Salad Deluxe	1	716	47	55	98	1419
Del Burger	1	385	20	35	42	1065
Del Cheeseburger	1	439	25	35	55	1268
Double Del Cheeseburger	1	618	39	36	108	1638
French Fries	1 lg serv	566	26	76	0	318
French Fries	1 reg serv	404	19	54	0	227
French Fries	1 sm serv	242	11	32	0	136
Fries, Chili Cheese	1 serv	562	30	58	38	846
Fries, Deluxe Chili Cheese	1 serv	600	33	61	48	855
Fries, Nacho	1 serv	669	34	80	2	926
Guacamole	1 oz	60	6	2	0	130
Hamburger	1	231	8	26	29	649
Hot Sauce	1 pkg	2	tr	tr	0	38

FOOD	PORTION	CAL	FAT	CARB	CHOL	SOD
Nacho Cheese Sauce Side Order	1 serv	100	8	4	2	401
Nachos	1 serv	390	32	39	2	504
Nachos Super Deluxe	1 serv	684	45	54	46	1469
Quesadilla	1	257	12	26	30	455
Quesadilla, Chicken	1	544	31	38	113	1147
Quesadilla, Regular	1	483	27	37	75	871
Salsa	2 oz	14	tr	3	tr	308
Salsa Dressing	1 oz	33	3	1	10	85
Sour Cream	1 oz	60	6	tr	20	15
Taco	1	140	8	10	16	99
Taco, Chicken	1	186	13	10	35	276
Taco, Deluxe Double Beef	1	205	13	13	35	159
Taco, Double Beef	1	172	10	12	25	150
Taco Salad	1	235	19	9	31	268
Taco Salad Deluxe	1	741	49	57	83	1280
Taco, Soft	1	146	6	17	16	223
Taco, Soft, Chicken	1	197	11	16	35	401
Taco, Soft, Deluxe Double Beef	1	211	11	20	35	283
Taco, Soft, Double Beef	1	178	8	18	25	274
Tostada	1	140	8	12	15	333

DENNY'S

BREAKFAST SELECTIONS

FOOD	PORTION	CAL	FAT	CARB	CHOL	SOD
Harvest Slam	1 serv	1050	55	—	44	2175
Harvest Slam w/ Egg Beaters	1 serv	960	46	—	33	2220
Omelette Chili Cheese	1 serv	490	33	—	230	1130

FOOD	PORTION	CAL	FAT	CARB	CHOL	SOD
Omelette *(cont.)*						
Denver	1 serv	720	62	—	650	890
Ham 'N' Cheddar	1 serv	480	33	—	240	1120
Mexican	1 serv	540	40	—	245	1060
Senior	1 serv	640	57	—	470	1340
Ultimate	1 serv	850	75	—	670	1220
Vegetable	1 serv	590	48	—	630	370
Vegetable w/ Egg Beaters	1 serv	450	34	—	15	430
Pancakes	3	410	6	—	—	1968
Senior Belgian Waffle Slam	1 serv	370	25	—	—	715
Senior Grand Slam Breakfast	1 serv	380	22	—	—	1050
Senior Starter w/ Bacon	1 serv	370	18	—	—	1110
Senior Starter w/ Sausage	1 serv	440	24	—	—	1220
DESSERTS						
Apple Pie, Regular	1 slice	480	26	—	4	260
Apple Pie w/ Equal	1 slice	460	30	—	0	200
MAIN MENU SELECTIONS						
Bacon Swiss w/o Lettuce & Tomato	1	750	45	—	130	1770
Baked Potato	1 med	90	0	—	0	7
BLT	1	620	38	—	40	1400
Carrots	1 serv (3 oz)	20	tr	—	—	30
Catfish	2 pieces (8 oz)	640	58	—	107	118
Chicken Fried Steak w/o Gravy	2 pieces	500	41	—	90	1500
Chicken Stir Fry w/ Rice	1 serv	420	20	—	60	970
Club Sandwich	1	590	34	—	90	1700

FOOD	PORTION	CAL	FAT	CARB	CHOL	SOD
Coleslaw	1 cup	120	10	—	—	150
Corn	1 serv (3 oz)	60	1	—	—	40
Denny Burger	1	490	24	—	70	790
French Fries	1 serv (4 oz)	300	16	—	—	70
Fried Chicken	4 pieces	460	30	—	—	1300
Green Beans	1 serv (3 oz)	15	tr	—	—	20
Grilled Cheese	1	710	48	—	100	2690
Grilled Chicken	1	520	26	—	60	950
Grilled Chicken Breast	1 serv	125	3	—	70	390
Ham & Swiss Sandwich	1	500	28	—	76	1620
Liver w/ Bacon & Onions	2 pieces	370	22	—	530	520
Mashed Potatoes	1 serv (4 oz)	70	tr	—	—	300
Onion Rings	1 ring	90	5	—	—	200
Patty Melt	1	775	57	—	120	1490
Peas	1 serv (3 oz)	40	tr	—	—	50
Quesadilla, Beef	1	730	48	—	100	2010
Quesadilla, Chicken	1	620	36	—	105	1890
Quesadilla, Denny's	1	510	33	—	45	1550
Rice Pilaf	⅓ cup	90	2	—	—	320
Senior Fried Shrimp w/o Vegetable or Bread	1 serv	330	13	—	—	1970
Senior Grilled Catfish Dinner	1 serv	320	29	—	—	60
Senior Grilled Chicken Breast Entree	1 serv	100	3	—	—	400
Senior Roast Beef Dinner w/o Vegetable	1 serv	280	9	—	80	520
Senior Roast Turkey & Stuffing Entree	1 serv	440	16	—	—	947

FOOD	PORTION	CAL	FAT	CARB	CHOL	SOD
Senior Sirloin Tips & Noodles	1 serv	220	5	—	—	680
Senior Spaghetti Dinner	1 serv	580	25	—	80	1010
Senior Turkey Sandwich	1 serv	340	27	—	—	1000
Stuffing	½ cup	180	9	—	—	400
Super Bird	1	750	37	—	110	2510
Top Sirloin Steak	1 serv	270	10	—	90	75
Tuna Sandwich	1	400	23	—	22	600
Turkey Sandwich	1	340	16	—	70	920
Turkey w/o Gravy	6 slices	200	6	—	120	1260
Veggie Cheese	1	560	40	—	70	1330
Veggie Cheese Melt	1	560	39	—	70	1330
Works Burger w/o Lettuce & Tomato	1	950	66	—	130	1360
SALADS AND SALAD BAR						
Chef Salad	1	370	26	—	320	1340
Garden Salad	1	110	4	—	75	160
Grilled Chicken Salad	1	290	12	—	80	90
Taco Salad	1	910	55	—	50	1860
SOUPS						
Cheese	1 serv	406	30	—	38	1740
Chicken Noodle	1 serv	120	4	—	20	1279
Cream of Potato	1 serv	250	9	—	—	1560
Vegetable Beef	1 serv	159	27	—	9	1640

DOMINO'S PIZZA

12-INCH PIZZA						
Pepperoni	1 slice	219	7	30	14	570
Veggie	1 slice	204	5	27	9	488
15-INCH PIZZA						
Deluxe	2 slices	498	20	59	40	954

FOOD	PORTION	CAL	FAT	CARB	CHOL	SOD
16-INCH PIZZA						
Cheese	2 slices	376	10	56	19	483
Double Cheese Pepperoni	2 slices	545	25	55	48	1042
Ham	2 slices	417	11	58	26	805
Pepperoni	2 slices	460	18	56	28	825
Sausage Mushroom	2 slices	430	16	55	28	552
Veggie	2 slices	498	19	60	36	1035

DUNKIN' DONUTS

FOOD	PORTION	CAL	FAT	CARB	CHOL	SOD
COOKIES						
Chocolate Chunk	1 (1.6 oz)	200	10	25	30	110
Chocolate Chunk w/ Nuts	1 (1.5 oz)	210	11	23	30	100
Oatmeal Pecan Raisin	1 (1.6 oz)	200	9	28	25	100
CROISSANTS						
Almond	1 (3.7 oz)	420	26	38	0	290
Chocolate	1 (3.3 oz)	440	29	38	0	240
Plain	1 (2.5 oz)	310	19	27	0	240
DONUTS						
Apple Crumb	1 (3 oz)	250	10	37	0	260
Apple Filled w/ Cinnamon Sugar	1 (2.8 oz)	250	11	33	0	280
Blueberry Filled	1 (2.4 oz)	210	8	29	0	240
Boston Kreme	1 (2.8 oz)	240	11	32	0	260
Butternut Cake Ring	1 (3.5 oz)	410	20	53	0	390
Chocolate Frosted Cake Ring	1 (2.3 oz)	280	16	28	0	330
Chocolate Frosted Yeast Ring	1 (1.9 oz)	200	10	25	0	190
Chocolate Glazed Ring	1 (3.4 oz)	420	24	46	0	410

FOOD	PORTION	CAL	FAT	CARB	CHOL	SOD
Chocolate Kreme	1 (2.4 oz)	250	14	28	0	210
Cinnamon Cake Ring	1 (2.2 oz)	260	15	27	0	340
Coconut Coated Cake Ring	1 (3.1 oz)	360	21	38	0	360
Dunkin' Donut	1 (2.1 oz)	240	14	26	0	370
Glazed Buttermilk Ring	1 (2.6 oz)	290	14	37	10	370
Glazed Chocolate Ring	1 (2.7 oz)	320	18	38	0	350
Glazed Coffee Roll	1 (2.8 oz)	280	12	37	0	310
Glazed Cruller	1 (2.4 oz)	260	11	36	0	330
Glazed French Cruller	1 (1.4 oz)	140	8	16	30	130
Glazed Whole Wheat Ring	1 (2.5 oz)	280	15	32	0	370
Glazed Yeast Ring	1 (1.9 oz)	200	9	26	0	230
Jelly Filled	1 (2.4 oz)	220	9	31	0	230
Lemon Filled	1 (2.8 oz)	260	12	33	0	280
Mini Cake	1 (0.9 oz)	100	6	10	0	142
Mini Chocolate Glazed	1 (1.1 oz)	122	7	14	0	169
Mini Cinnamon Cake	1 (1 oz)	116	7	12	0	151
Mini Coconut	1 (1.2 oz)	140	8	15	0	140
Mini Coffee Roll	1 (0.8 oz)	78	3	11	0	87
Mini Eclairs	1 (1.3 oz)	114	5	15	0	122
Munchkin Butternut Cake	1 (0.6 oz)	70	3	10	0	70
Munchkin Coconut Cake	1 (0.6 oz)	70	4	8	0	80
Munchkin Glazed Cake	1 (0.6 oz)	60	3	9	0	70
Munchkin Glazed Chocolate	1 (0.7 oz)	70	3	10	0	90
Munchkin Glazed Yeast	1 (0.5 oz)	50	2	7	0	40

FOOD	PORTION	CAL	FAT	CARB	CHOL	SOD
Munchkin Jelly Filled Yeast	1 (0.5 oz)	50	2	7	0	40
Munchkin Plain Cake	1 (0.5 oz)	50	3	6	0	70
Munchkin Powdered Cake	1 (0.5 oz)	50	3	6	0	70
Peanut	1 (3.7 oz)	480	29	44	0	350
Plain Cake Ring	1 (2 oz)	262	18	23	0	330
Powdered Cake Ring	1 (2.2 oz)	270	16	28	0	340
Sugared Cake Ring	1 (2.1 oz)	270	18	25	0	320
Sugared Jelly Stick	1 (3 oz)	310	12	46	0	380
Vanilla Frosted Yeast Ring	1 (2 oz)	200	9	26	0	220
Vanilla Kreme	1 (2.4 oz)	250	12	31	0	250
MUFFINS						
Apple N'Spice	1 (3.4 oz)	300	8	52	25	360
Banana Nut	1 (3.3 oz)	310	10	49	30	410
Blueberry	1 (3.6 oz)	280	8	46	30	340
Bran w/ Raisins	1 (3.68 oz)	310	9	51	15	560
Corn	1 (3.4 oz)	340	12	51	40	560
Cranberry Nut	1 (3.4 oz)	290	9	44	25	360
Oat Bran	1 (3.3 oz)	330	11	50	0	450

EL POLLO LOCO

FOOD	PORTION	CAL	FAT	CARB	CHOL	SOD
DESSERTS						
Cheesecake	1 serv (3.5 oz)	160	18	30	60	230
Churros	1 serv (1.5 oz)	140	9	14	4	180
Orange Bang	1 serv (7 oz)	110	0	26	0	24
Pina Colada Bang	1 serv (7 oz)	110	0	26	0	24
MAIN MENU SELECTIONS						
Beans	1 serv (4 oz)	100	3	16	0	460
Burrito, Chicken	1 (7 oz)	310	11	30	65	510
Burrito, Steak	1 (6 oz)	450	22	31	70	740

FOOD	PORTION	CAL	FAT	CARB	CHOL	SOD
Burrito, Vegetarian	1 (6 oz)	340	7	54	20	360
Cheddar Cheese	1 serv (1 oz)	90	5	3	27	180
Chicken Breast	1 (3 oz)	160	6	0	110	390
Chicken Fajita Meal	1 (17.5 oz)	780	18	130	58	1060
Chicken Leg	1 (1.75 oz)	90	5	0	75	150
Chicken Thigh	1 (2 oz)	180	12	0	130	230
Chicken Wing	1 (1.5 oz)	110	6	0	80	220
Coleslaw	1 serv (3 oz)	70	8	7	0	350
Corn	1 serv (3 oz)	110	2	20	0	110
Guacamole	1 serv (1 oz)	60	6	2	0	130
Potato Salad	1 serv (4 oz)	180	10	21	10	340
Rice	1 serv (2 oz)	110	2	19	0	220
Salsa	2 oz	10	0	3	0	180
Sour Cream	1 serv (1 oz)	60	6	1	13	15
Steak Fajita Meal	1 (17.5 oz)	1040	38	120	100	1550
Taco, Chicken	1 (5 oz)	180	7	18	35	300
Taco, Steak	1 (4.5 oz)	250	12	18	40	410
Tortillas, Corn	1 (1 oz)	60	1	13	0	25
Tortillas, Flour	1 (1 oz)	90	3	15	0	150
SALAD DRESSINGS						
Blue Cheese	1 oz	80	6	4	5	150
Deluxe French	1 oz	60	4	7	0	160
Honey Dijon Mustard	1 oz	50	1	7	0	440
Italian Reduced Calorie	1 oz	25	2	2	0	170
Ranch	1 oz	75	6	4	0	190
Thousand Island	1 oz	110	10	4	5	240
SALADS AND SALAD BAR						
Chicken Salad	1 (12 oz)	160	4	11	45	440
Side Salad	1 (9 oz)	50	1	10	0	30

FOOD	PORTION	CAL	FAT	CARB	CHOL	SOD
GODFATHER'S PIZZA						
Golden Crust Cheese	⅒ lg (3.5 oz)	261	11	31	23	314
Golden Crust Cheese	⅛ med (3.1 oz)	229	9	28	19	272
Golden Crust Cheese	⅙ sm (3 oz)	213	8	27	19	258
Golden Crust Combo	⅒ lg (5.1 oz)	322	15	33	34	602
Golden Crust Combo	⅛ med (4.5 oz)	283	13	30	29	526
Golden Crust Combo	⅙ sm (4.5 oz)	273	12	29	31	542
Golden Crust Combo	⅙ sm (4.5 oz)	273	12	29	31	542
Original Crust Cheese	⅒ lg (4 oz)	271	8	37	28	329
Original Crust Cheese	⅛ med (3.5 oz)	242	7	35	22	285
Original Crust Cheese	¼ mini (2 oz)	138	4	20	13	159
Original Crust Cheese	⅙ sm (3.5 oz)	239	7	32	25	289
Original Crust Combo	⅒ lg (5.5 oz)	332	12	39	39	617
Original Crust Combo	⅛ med (5.2 oz)	318	12	37	38	569
Original Crust Combo	¼ mini (2.8 oz)	164	5	21	17	287
Original Crust Combo	⅙ sm (5 oz)	299	11	34	37	573
HAAGEN-DAZS						
FROZEN YOGURT						
Banana, Nonfat Soft	1 oz	25	0	5	0	15
Chocolate	3 oz	130	3	21	25	30
Chocolate, Nonfat Soft	1 oz	30	0	6	0	20
Chocolate, Soft	1 oz	30	1	4	3	15
Coffee, Soft	1 oz	28	1	4	3	13
Peach	3 oz	120	3	20	31	30
Raspberry, Soft	1 oz	30	1	5	3	15
Strawberry	3 oz	120	3	21	30	30
Strawberry, Nonfat Soft	1 oz	25	0	5	0	10
Vanilla	3 oz	130	3	20	40	40

FOOD	PORTION	CAL	FAT	CARB	CHOL	SOD
Vanilla Almond Crunch	3 oz	150	5	22	33	65
Vanilla, Soft	1 oz	28	1	4	3	13
ICE CREAM Butter Pecan	4 oz	390	24	29	115	100
Caramel Almond Crunch Bar	1	240	18	17	40	65
Caramel Nut Sundae	4 oz	310	21	26	—	100
Chocolate	4 oz	270	17	24	120	50
Chocolate Chocolate Chip	4 oz	290	20	28	105	40
Chocolate Chocolate Mint	4 oz	300	20	26	—	50
Chocolate Dark Chocolate Bar	1	390	27	32	—	60
Coffee	4 oz	270	17	23	120	55
Deep Chocolate	4 oz	290	14	26	—	70
Deep Chocolate Fudge	4 oz	290	14	26	—	90
Honey Vanilla	4 oz	250	16	22	135	55
Macadamia Brittle	4 oz	280	18	25	—	60
Orange & Cream Pop	1	130	6	18	—	25
Peanut Butter Crunch Bar	1 (6.3 fl oz)	270	21	16	35	55
Rum Raisin	4 oz	250	17	21	110	45
Strawberry	4 oz	250	15	23	95	40
Vanilla	4 oz	260	17	23	120	55
Vanilla Crunch Bar	1	220	16	16	40	55
Vanilla Fudge	4 oz	270	17	26	—	100
Vanilla Milk Chocolate Almond Bar	1	370	27	27	—	55
Vanilla Milk Chocolate Bar	1	360	27	26	—	55

FOOD	PORTION	CAL	FAT	CARB	CHOL	SOD
Vanilla Milk Chocolate Brittle Bar	1	370	25	32	—	160
Vanilla Peanut Butter Swirl	4 oz	280	21	19	110	120
Vanilla Swiss Almond	4 oz	290	19	24	—	55
ICES AND ICE POPS						
Blueberry Sorbet & Cream	4 oz	190	8	25	—	35
Fudge Pop Bar	1	210	14	19	—	50
Key Lime Sorbet & Cream	4 oz	190	7	29	—	30
Lemon Sorbet	4 oz	140	0	34	—	5
Orange Sorbet	4 oz	113	0	30	—	7
Orange Sorbet & Cream	4 oz	190	8	27	—	35
Raspberry Sorbet	4 oz	93	0	22	—	7
Raspberry Sorbet & Cream	4 oz	180	8	23	—	35

HARDEE'S

BAKED SELECTIONS						
Big Cookie	1 (2.0 oz)	280	12	41	15	150
Blueberry Muffin	1 (4 oz)	400	17	56	65	310
BEVERAGES						
Orange Juice	1 serv (11 oz)	140	tr	34	0	5
Shake, Chocolate	1 (11.4 fl oz)	390	10	61	30	220
Shake, Peach	1 (11.4 fl oz)	530	11	95	45	220
Shake, Strawberry	1 (11.4 fl oz)	390	8	65	30	200
Shake, Vanilla	1 (11.4 fl oz)	370	9	59	25	210
BREAKFAST SELECTIONS						
Bacon & Egg Biscuit	1 (4.4 oz)	490	27	44	155	1250
Bacon, Egg & Cheese Biscuit	1 (4.8 oz)	530	31	45	155	1470
Big Country Breakfast w/ Bacon	1 (7.6 oz)	740	43	61	305	1800

FOOD	PORTION	CAL	FAT	CARB	CHOL	SOD
Big Country Breakfast w/ Sausage	1 (9.6 oz)	930	61	61	340	2240
Biscuit 'N' Gravy	1 (7.8 oz)	510	28	55	15	1500
Canadian Rise 'N' Shine Biscuit	1 (5.8 oz)	570	32	46	175	1860
Chicken Biscuit	1 (5.1 oz)	510	25	52	45	1580
Cinnamon 'N' Raisin Biscuit	1 (2.8 oz)	370	18	48	0	450
Country Ham Biscuit	1 (3.8 oz)	430	22	45	25	1930
Frisco Breakfast Ham Sandwich	1 (6.5 oz)	460	22	46	175	1320
Ham Biscuit	1 (4 oz)	400	20	47	15	1340
Ham, Egg & Cheese Biscuit	1 (5.6 oz)	500	27	48	170	1620
Hash Rounds	1 serv (2.8 oz)	230	14	24	0	560
Rise 'N' Shine Biscuit	1 (2.9 oz)	390	21	44	0	1000
Sausage & Egg Biscuit	1 (5.2 oz)	560	35	44	170	1400
Sausage Biscuit	1 (4.1 oz)	510	31	44	25	1360
Steak Biscuit	1 (5.2 oz)	580	32	56	30	1580
Three Pancakes	1 serv (4.8 oz)	280	2	56	15	890
Three Pancakes w/ 1 Sausage Patty	1 serv (6.2 oz)	430	16	56	40	1290
Three Pancakes w/ 2 Bacon Strips	1 serv (5.3 oz)	350	9	56	25	1130
ICE CREAM						
Cool Twist Sundae, Hot Fudge	1 (5.9 oz)	320	10	50	25	260
Cool Twist Sundae, Strawberry	1 (5.8 oz)	260	6	48	15	100
Cool Twist Cone, Chocolate	1 (4.1 oz)	180	4	29	15	85
Cool Twist Cone, Vanilla	1 (4.1 oz)	180	4	29	15	80

FOOD	PORTION	CAL	FAT	CARB	CHOL	SOD
Cool Twist Cone, Vanilla/Chocolate	1 (4.1 oz)	170	4	29	15	85

MAIN MENU SELECTIONS

FOOD	PORTION	CAL	FAT	CARB	CHOL	SOD
Bacon Cheeseburger	1 (7.9 oz)	600	36	35	50	950
Big Deluxe Burger	1 (8.5 oz)	530	30	36	40	790
Big Roast Beef Sandwich	1 (5.9 oz)	370	16	34	40	1050
Cheeseburger	1 (4.2 oz)	300	13	34	25	690
Chef Salad	1 (9.4 oz)	200	13	5	45	910
Chicken Fillet Sandwich	1 (6.6 oz)	400	14	48	55	1100
Coleslaw	1 serv (4 oz)	240	20	13	10	340
Crispy Curls	1 serv (3.0 oz)	300	16	36	0	840
Fisherman's Fillet Sandwich	1 (7.6 oz)	500	22	51	60	1170
French Fries	1 lg serv (6.1 oz)	430	18	59	0	190
French Fries	1 med serv (5.0 oz)	350	15	49	0	150
French Fries	1 sm serv (3.4 oz)	240	10	33	0	100
Fried Chicken Breast	1 (5.2 oz)	370	15	29	75	1190
Fried Chicken Leg	1 (2.4 oz)	170	7	15	45	570
Fried Chicken Thigh	1 (4.2 oz)	330	15	30	60	1000
Fried Chicken Wing	1 (2.3 oz)	200	8	23	30	740
Frisco Burger	1 (8.5 oz)	760	50	43	70	1280
Frisco Grilled Chicken Sandwich	1 (8.6 oz)	620	34	44	95	1730
Garden Salad	1 (9.3 oz)	190	14	3	40	280
Gravy	1 serv (1.5 fl oz)	20	tr	3	0	260
Grilled Chicken Salad	1 (9.8 oz)	120	4	2	60	520
Hamburger	1 (3.6 oz)	260	9	33	20	460
Hot Dog	1 (6.8 oz)	450	20	52	35	1090

FOOD	PORTION	CAL	FAT	CARB	CHOL	SOD
Hot Ham 'N' Cheese Sandwich	1 (7.1 oz)	530	30	49	65	1710
Mashed Potatoes	1 serv (4 oz)	70	tr	14	0	330
Mushroom 'N' Swiss Burger	1 (7.1 oz)	520	27	37	45	990
Quarter-Pound Cheeseburger	1 (6.5 oz)	490	25	37	35	860
Regular Roast Beef Sandwich	1 (4.4 oz)	270	11	28	25	780
Side Salad	1 (4.9 oz)	20	tr	3	0	20

H-SALT SEAFOOD

FOOD	PORTION	CAL	FAT	CARB	CHOL	SOD
Chicken	3 oz	108	6	—	69	2
Cod	3 oz	62	2	—	18	57
Hamburger	3 oz	228	18	—	65	40
Pork Loin	3 oz	254	21	—	55	55
Sirloin Steak	3 oz	239	20	—	58	36

IHOP

FOOD	PORTION	CAL	FAT	CARB	CHOL	SOD
Buckwheat Pancake	1 (2.5 oz)	134	5	19	61	372
Buttermilk Pancake	1 (2 oz)	108	3	17	31	459
Egg Pancake	1 (2 oz)	102	5	12	66	213
Harvest Grain 'N Nut Pancake	1 (2.25 oz)	160	8	18	38	391
Waffle	1 (4 oz)	305	15	37	70	468
Belgian Waffle	1 (6 oz)	408	20	49	146	882
Belgian Harvest Grain 'N Nut Waffle	1 (6 oz)	445	28	40	147	876

JACK IN THE BOX

BEVERAGES

FOOD	PORTION	CAL	FAT	CARB	CHOL	SOD
Coca-Cola Classic	1 sm (16 fl oz)	190	0	48	0	20

FOOD	PORTION	CAL	FAT	CARB	CHOL	SOD
Coffee, Black	1 cup (8 fl oz)	0	0	0	0	25
Diet Coke	1 sm (16 fl oz)	0	0	0	0	35
Dr Pepper	1 sm (16 fl oz)	190	0	49	0	25
Iced Tea	1 sm (16 fl oz)	5	0	tr	0	5
Milk, 2%	1 serv (8 oz)	120	5	12	20	120
Milk Shake, Chocolate	1 reg (11 fl oz)	330	7	55	25	270
Milk Shake, Strawberry	1 reg (11 fl oz)	320	7	55	25	240
Milk Shake, Vanilla	1 reg (11 fl oz)	320	6	57	25	230
Orange Juice	1 serv (6 fl oz)	80	0	20	0	0
Ramblin' Root Beer	1 sm (16 fl oz)	240	0	61	0	30
Sprite	1 sm (16 fl oz)	190	0	48	0	60

BREAKFAST SELECTIONS

FOOD	PORTION	CAL	FAT	CARB	CHOL	SOD
Breakfast Jack	1 (4.4 oz)	310	13	30	200	870
Country Crock Spread	1 pat (5 g)	25	3	0	0	40
Grape Jelly	1 serv (0.5 oz)	40	0	9	0	5
Hash Browns	1 serv (2 oz)	160	11	14	0	310
Pancake Platter	1 (8.1 oz)	610	22	87	87	390
Pancake Syrup	1 serv (1.5 fl oz)	120	0	30	0	5
Sausage Crescent	1 (5.5 oz)	580	43	28	185	1010
Scrambled Egg Platter	1 (7.5 oz)	560	32	50	380	1060
Scrambled Egg Pocket	1 (6.4 oz)	430	21	31	355	1060
Sourdough Breakfast Sandwich	1 (5.2 oz)	380	20	31	235	1120
Supreme Crescent	1 (5.1 oz)	550	40	27	180	1050

DESSERTS

FOOD	PORTION	CAL	FAT	CARB	CHOL	SOD
Cheesecake	1 serv (3.5 oz)	310	18	29	65	210
Cinnamon Churritos	1 serv (2.6 oz)	330	21	34	20	200
Double Fudge Cake	1 slice (3 oz)	290	9	49	20	260
Hot Apple Turnover	1 (3.9 oz)	350	19	48	0	50

FOOD	PORTION	CAL	FAT	CARB	CHOL	SOD
MAIN MENU SELECTIONS						
Bacon Bacon Cheeseburger	1 (8.5 oz)	710	45	41	110	1240
Barbeque Sauce	1 serv (1 oz)	45	tr	11	0	300
Beef Gyro	1 (9.1 oz)	620	32	55	65	1310
Buttermilk House Sauce	1 serv (0.9 oz)	130	13	3	5	240
Cheeseburger	1 (3.9 oz)	320	14	33	40	750
Chicken & Mushroom Sandwich	1 (7.8 oz)	440	18	40	61	1340
Chicken Fajita Pita	1 (6.6 oz)	290	8	29	35	700
Chicken Sandwich	1 (5.6 oz)	400	18	38	45	1290
Chicken Strips	6 pieces (6.2 oz)	450	20	28	80	1100
Chicken Strips	4 pieces (3.9 oz)	290	13	18	50	700
Chicken Supreme	1 (8.6 oz)	670	42	48	75	1520
Chimichangas, Mini	4 pieces (7.3 oz)	570	28	57	65	630
Chimichangas, Mini	6 pieces (10.9 oz)	860	42	85	95	950
Country Fried Steak Sandwich	1 (5.4 oz)	450	25	42	35	890
Double Cheeseburger	1 (5.2 oz)	470	27	33	70	840
Egg Rolls	5 pieces (10 oz)	750	41	92	50	1640
Egg Rolls	3 pieces (5.5 oz)	440	24	54	30	960
Fish Supreme	1 (8.6 oz)	590	32	15	60	1170
French Fries	1 jumbo serv (4.3 oz)	400	19	51	0	220
French Fries	1 reg serv (3.8 oz)	350	17	45	0	190
French Fries	1 sm serv (2.4 oz)	220	11	28	0	120
Grilled Chicken Fillet	1 (7.4 oz)	430	19	36	65	1070
Grilled Sourdough Burger	1 (7.8 oz)	710	50	34	110	1140

FOOD	PORTION	CAL	FAT	CARB	CHOL	SOD
Guacamole	1 serv (0.9 oz)	30	3	2	0	130
Hamburger	1 (3.4 oz)	270	11	28	25	560
Hot Sauce	1 serv (0.5 oz)	5	0	1	0	110
Jumbo Jack	1 (7.8 oz)	580	34	42	70	730
Jumbo Jack w/ Cheese	1 (8.9 oz)	680	40	46	100	1090
Onion Rings	1 serv (3.6 oz)	380	23	38	0	450
Quarter-Pound Burger	1 (6 oz)	510	27	39	65	1030
Salsa	1 serv (1 oz)	10	tr	2	0	30
Seasoned Curly French Fries	1 serv (3.8 oz)	360	20	39	0	1030
Sesame Breadsticks	1 (0.6 oz)	70	2	12	0	110
Sirloin Steak Sandwich	1 (8.3 oz)	520	23	49	65	1050
Smoked Chicken, Cheddar & Bacon Sandwich	1 (7.8 oz)	540	30	37	80	1520
Spicy Crispy Chicken Sandwich	1 (7.8 oz)	560	27	55	50	1020
Super Taco	1 (4.4 oz)	280	17	22	30	720
Sweet & Sour Sauce	1 serv (1 oz)	40	tr	11	0	160
Taco	1 (2.7 oz)	190	11	15	20	410
Teriyaki Bowl, Beef	1 serv (15.4 oz)	640	3	124	25	930
Teriyaki Bowl, Chicken	1 serv (15.4 oz)	580	2	115	30	1220
Tortilla Chips	1 serv (1 oz)	140	6	18	0	135
Ultimate Cheeseburger	1 (9.8 oz)	940	69	33	130	1180
SALAD DRESSINGS Bleu Cheese	1 serv (2.5 oz)	260	22	14	20	920
Buttermilk House	1 serv (2.5 oz)	360	36	8	20	690
Italian Low Calorie	1 serv (2.5 oz)	25	2	2	0	810
Thousand Island	1 serv (2.5 oz)	310	30	12	25	700

FOOD	PORTION	CAL	FAT	CARB	CHOL	SOD
SALADS AND SALAD BAR						
Chef Salad	1 (11.4 oz)	320	19	9	130	930
Side Salad	1 (4 oz)	50	3	tr	0	85
Taco Salad	1 (14.1 oz)	500	31	28	90	1600

KENTUCKY FRIED CHICKEN

FOOD	PORTION	CAL	FAT	CARB	CHOL	SOD
BAKED SELECTIONS						
Biscuit	1 (2.2 oz)	220	12	26	<5	530
Breakstick	1 (1.2 oz)	110	3	17	0	15
Cornbread	1 (2 oz)	228	13	25	42	194
Sourdough Roll	1 (1.7 oz)	128	2	24	0	236
MAIN MENU SELECTIONS						
BBQ Baked Beans	1 serv (3.9 oz)	132	2	24	3	535
Chicken Littles Sandwich	1 (1.7 oz)	169	10	14	18	331
Coleslaw	1 serv (3.2 oz)	114	6	13	<5	177
Colonel's Chicken Sandwich	1 (5.9 oz)	482	27	39	47	1060
Colonel's Rotisserie Gold						
Dark Quarter	1 serv (5.1 oz)	333	24	1	163	980
Dark Quarter, Skin Removed	1 serv (4.1 oz)	217	12	0	128	772
White Quarter	1 serv (6.2 oz)	335	19	1	157	1104
White Quarter, Skin Removed	1 serv (4.1 oz)	199	6	0	97	667
Corn on the Cob	1 ear (5.3 oz)	222	12	27	0	76
Crispy Fries	1 serv (2.5 oz)	210	11	24	4	493
Extra Tasty						
Crispy Center Breast	1 (4.1 oz)	330	19	14	75	740
Crispy Drumstick	1 (2.3 oz)	190	12	6	65	310
Crispy Side Breast	1 (4.1 oz)	400	27	19	75	710

FOOD	PORTION	CAL	FAT	CARB	CHOL	SOD
Crispy Thigh	1 (3.8 oz)	380	29	7	90	520
Crispy Whole Wing	1 (2.1 oz)	240	17	8	65	440
Garden Rice	1 serv (3.8 oz)	75	1	15	0	576
Green Beans	1 serv (3.6 oz)	36	1	5	3	563
Hot & Spicy						
Center Breast	1 (4.3 oz)	360	22	13	80	750
Drumstick	1 (2.4 oz)	180	12	6	55	320
Side Breast	1 (4.2 oz)	400	28	16	80	850
Thigh	1 (4.2 oz)	370	27	10	100	670
Whole Wing	1 (2.1 oz)	220	16	5	65	440
Hot Wings	6 (4.8 oz)	471	33	18	150	1230
Kentucky Nuggets	6 (3.4 oz)	284	18	15	66	865
Macaroni & Cheese	1 serv (4 oz)	162	8	15	16	531
Mashed Potatoes w/ Gravy	1 serv (4.2 oz)	70	1	15	<5	370
Mean Greens	1 serv (3.9 oz)	52	2	8	6	477
Original						
Center Breast	1 (3.6 oz)	260	14	8	92	609
Drumstick	1 (2 oz)	152	9	3	75	269
Side Breast	1 (2.9 oz)	245	15	9	78	604
Thigh	1 (3.4 oz)	287	21	8	112	591
Whole Wing	1 (1.9 oz)	172	11	5	59	383
Potato Wedges	1 serv (3.3 oz)	192	9	25	3	428
Red Beans & Rice	1 serv (3.9 oz)	114	3	18	4	315
Vegetable Medley Salad	1 serv (4 oz)	126	4	21	0	240
SALAD DRESSINGS						
Italian	1 serv (1 oz)	15	1	2	0	420
Ranch	1 serv (1 oz)	170	18	1	10	250
SALADS AND SALAD BAR						
Garden Salad	1 (3.1 oz)	16	0	3	0	10

FOOD	PORTION	CAL	FAT	CARB	CHOL	SOD
Macaroni Salad	1 serv (3.8 oz)	248	17	20	12	6
Pasta Salad	1 serv (3.8 oz)	135	8	14	1	663
Potato Salad	1 serv (4.4 oz)	180	11	18	11	423

KRYSTAL

BEVERAGES
Chocolate Shake	1 (12.8 fl oz)	271	10	41	32	175

BREAKFAST SELECTIONS
Biscuit	1 (3.2 oz)	289	14	35	1	777
Biscuit, Bacon	1 (3.6 oz)	355	20	36	14	1055
Biscuit, Country Ham	1 (4.5 oz)	379	19	36	23	1488
Biscuit, Egg	1 (4.8 oz)	372	21	36	133	813
Biscuit Gravy	1 (8.2 oz)	445	26	43	13	1306
Biscuit, Sausage	1 (4.3 oz)	429	27	37	29	987
Sunriser	1 (3.6 oz)	264	17	17	157	551

DESSERTS
Apple Pie	1 serv (4.5 oz)	320	14	45	0	420
Donut	1 (1.3 oz)	100	9	17	6	130
Donut w/ Chocolate Icing	1 (1.8 oz)	162	11	27	6	149
Donut w/ Vanilla Icing	1 (1.8 oz)	148	9	29	6	130
Lemon Meringue Pie	1 serv (4 oz)	340	9	60	45	130
Pecan Pie	1 serv (4 oz)	450	24	61	55	290

MAIN MENU SELECTIONS
Bacon Cheeseburger	1 (6.4 oz)	583	35	34	114	935
Big K	1 (7.3 oz)	608	36	35	125	1281
Burger Plus	1 (6.4 oz)	488	27	36	90	709
Burger Plus w/ Cheese	1 (7 oz)	545	31	37	105	962
Cheese Krystal	1 (2.6 oz)	189	10	16	30	456
Chicken Sandwich	1 (6.4 oz)	392	16	44	33	707
Chili	1 lg (12 oz)	322	11	33	25	1012

FOOD	PORTION	CAL	FAT	CARB	CHOL	SOD
Chili	1 reg (8 oz)	214	8	22	16	674
Chili Cheese Pup	1 (2.6 oz)	203	13	15	24	623
Chili Pup	1 (2.5 oz)	184	12	14	19	593
Corn Pup	1 (2.3 oz)	214	14	17	24	566
Double Cheese Krystal	1 (4.6 oz)	341	19	25	60	824
Double Krystal	1 (4 oz)	276	14	24	43	532
Fries	1 lg serv (5 oz)	615	17	111	15	191
Fries	1 med serv (3.9 oz)	474	13	86	12	147
Fries	1 sm serv (2.8 oz)	338	9	61	8	105
Krys Kross Fries	1 serv (2.6 oz)	242	11	33	10	589
Krystal	1 (2.2 oz)	157	7	16	21	310
Plain Pup	1 (1.9 oz)	164	10	14	15	469

LITTLE CAESARS PIZZA

FOOD	PORTION	CAL	FAT	CARB	CHOL	SOD
Antipasto Salad	1 sm	96	5	8	10	320
Crazy Bread	1 piece	98	1	18	2	119
Crazy Sauce	1 serv	63	1	11	0	360
Greek Salad	1 sm	85	5	6	10	400
Ham & Cheese Sandwich	1	552	27	47	50	1580
Italian Sandwich	1	615	35	47	55	1580
Tossed Salad	1 sm	37	1	7	0	85
Tuna Sandwich	1	610	31	51	75	1080
Turkey Sandwich	1	450	17	49	45	1590
Veggie Sandwich	1	784	47	48	95	920
PIZZA Baby Pan!Pan!	1 order	525	22	53	60	1180
Cheese & Pepperoni Round, Large	1 slice	185	7	18	20	300

FOOD	PORTION	CAL	FAT	CARB	CHOL	SOD
Cheese & Pepperoni *(cont.)*						
Round, Medium	1 slice	168	7	16	20	270
Round, Small	1 slice	151	6	14	15	240
Square, Large	1 slice	204	8	22	25	430
Square, Medium	1 slice	201	8	22	23	430
Square, Small	1 slice	204	8	22	20	435
Cheese						
Round, Large	1 slice	169	6	18	15	240
Round, Medium	1 slice	154	5	16	15	220
Round, Small	1 slice	138	5	14	15	200
Square, Large	1 slice	188	6	22	20	380
Square, Medium	1 slice	185	6	22	20	370
Square, Small	1 slice	188	6	22	20	380
Slice! Slice!	1 order	756	31	71	90	1260

LONG JOHN SILVER'S

CHILDREN'S MENU SELECTIONS

FOOD	PORTION	CAL	FAT	CARB	CHOL	SOD
1 Fish, 1 Chicken & Fries	1 meal (8.9 oz)	620	34	61	45	1400
1 Piece Fish & Fries	1 meal (7 oz)	500	28	50	50	1010
2 Chicken Planks & Fries	1 meal (7.8 oz)	560	29	60	30	1310
DESSERTS						
Apple Pie	1 slice (4.5 oz)	320	13	45	—	420
Cherry Pie	1 slice (4.5 oz)	360	13	55	5	200
Chocolate Chip Cookie	1 (1.8 oz)	230	9	35	10	35
Lemon Pie	1 slice (4 oz)	340	9	60	45	130
Oatmeal Raisin Cookie	1 (1.8 oz)	160	10	15	15	150
Pineapple Cream Cheese Cake	1 slice (3.2 oz)	310	18	34	10	105
Walnut Brownie	1 (3.4 oz)	440	22	54	20	150

FOOD	PORTION	CAL	FAT	CARB	CHOL	SOD
MAIN MENU SELECTIONS						
Baked Chicken Entree	1 dinner (15.9 oz)	590	15	82	75	1620
Baked Chicken Light Herb	1 piece (3.5 oz)	120	4	tr	60	570
Baked Fish w/ Lemon Crumb	3 pieces (5 oz)	150	1	4	110	370
Baked Light Fish w/ Lemon Crumb Entree, 2 Pieces	1 dinner (11.8 oz)	330	5	46	46	640
Baked Fish w/ Lemon Crumb Entree, 3 Pieces	1 dinner (17.4 oz)	610	13	86	125	1420
Batter-Dipped Fish	1 piece (3.1 oz)	180	11	12	30	490
Batter-Dipped Shrimp	1 piece (0.4 oz)	30	2	2	10	80
Chicken Plank	1 piece (2 oz)	120	6	11	15	400
Chicken Planks	2 pieces (4 oz)	240	12	22	30	790
Chicken Planks, 2 Pieces & Fries	1 serv (6.9 oz)	490	26	50	30	1290
Chicken Planks, 3 Pieces w/ Fries & Slaw	1 serv (14.1 oz)	890	44	101	55	2000
Clams w/ Fries & Slaw	1 serv (12.7 oz)	990	52	114	75	1830
Coleslaw	1 serv (3.4 oz)	140	6	20	15	260
Corn Cobbette	1 piece (3.3 oz)	140	8	18	0	0
Crispy Fish	1 piece (1.8 oz)	150	8	8	20	240
Crispy Fish & More, 3 Pieces w/ Fries & Slaw	1 serv (13.5 oz)	980	50	92	70	1530
1 Fish, 1 Chicken & Fries	1 serv (8.1 oz)	550	32	51	45	1380
1 Fish & 2 Chicken w/ Fries & Slaw	1 serv (15.2 oz)	950	49	102	75	2090

FOOD	PORTION	CAL	FAT	CARB	CHOL	SOD
2 Fish, 4 Shrimp Clams w/ Fries & Slaw	1 serv (18.1 oz)	1240	70	123	140	2630
2 Fish, 5 Shrimp, 1 Chicken w/ Fries & Slaw	1 serv (18.1 oz)	1160	65	113	135	2590
2 Fish, 8 Shrimp w/ Fries & Slaw	1 serv (17.2 oz)	1140	65	108	145	2440
Fish & Fries, 2 Pieces	1 serv (9.2 oz)	610	37	52	52	1480
Fish & More, 2 Pieces w/ Fries & Slaw	1 serv (14.4 oz)	890	48	92	75	1790
Fries	1 serv (3 oz)	250	15	28	0	500
Green Beans	1 serv (3.5 oz)	20	tr	3	0	320
Honey Mustard Sauce	1 serv (0.42 oz)	20	tr	5	0	60
Hushpuppies	1 (0.8 oz)	70	2	10	<5	25
Ketchup	1 serv (.32 oz)	12	0	2	0	135
Rice	1 serv (4 oz)	190	4	36	0	300
Roll	1 (1.5 oz)	110	tr	23	0	170
Saltine Crackers	1 pkg (0.2 oz)	25	1	4	0	75
Sandwich, Batter Dipped Chicken, 1 Piece	1 (4.5 oz)	280	8	39	15	790
Sandwich, Batter Dipped fish, 1 Piece	1 (5.6 oz)	340	13	40	30	890
Seafood Sauce	1 serv (0.42 oz)	14	tr	3	0	180
Shrimp Scampi	10.6 oz	610	18	87	220	2050
Sweet 'N Sour Sauce	1 serv (0.42 oz)	20	tr	5	0	45
Tartar Sauce	1 serv (0.42 oz)	50	5	2	0	35
SALAD DRESSINGS						
Creamy Italian	1 serv (1 oz)	30	3	tr	—	280
Malt Vinegar	1 serv (0.28 oz)	1	tr	0	0	15
Ranch	1 serv (1 oz)	180	19	tr	<5	230

FOOD	PORTION	CAL	FAT	CARB	CHOL	SOD
Sea Salad	1 serv (1 oz)	140	15	2	<5	160
SALADS AND SALAD BAR						
Ocean Chef Salad	1 serv (8.3 oz)	110	1	13	40	730
Seafood Salad	1 serv (9.8 oz)	380	31	12	55	980
Side Salad	1 (4.4 oz)	25	tr	6	0	20
SOUPS						
Seafood Chowder w/ Cod	1 serv (7 oz)	140	6	10	20	590
Seafood Gumbo w/ Cod	1 serv (7 oz)	120	8	4	25	740

MACHEEZMO MOUSE

FOOD	PORTION	CAL	FAT	CARB	CHOL	SOD
CHILDREN'S MENU SELECTIONS						
Kid's Plate	7 oz	279	5	44	20	328
Kid's Plate w/ Chicken	9 oz	349	7	44	80	358
MAIN MENU SELECTIONS						
Bean & Cheese Enchilada	12 oz	405	8	63	28	450
Bean & Cheese Enchilada Dinner	22 oz	670	8	121	28	710
Beans	6 oz	214	0	42	0	120
Boss Sauce	1 oz	30	0	8	0	140
Cheese	1 oz	81	5	1	20	180
Cheese Quesadilla	5 oz	337	13	35	42	535
Chicken	3 oz	105	3	0	90	45
Chicken Burrito	13 oz	543	10	76	110	653
Chicken Burrito Dinner	23 oz	808	10	135	110	913
Chicken Enchilada	10 oz	332	10	35	88	400
Chicken Enchilada Dinner	20 oz	597	10	93	88	660
Chicken Majita	18 oz	704	9	121	128	784
Chicken Quesadilla	9 oz	407	15	35	102	575

FOOD	PORTION	CAL	FAT	CARB	CHOL	SOD
Chicken Salad, Large	17 oz	612	15	84	122	750
Chicken Salad, Small	10 oz	324	75	45	76	390
Chicken Tacos	6 oz	294	8	31	82	255
Chicken Tacos Dinner	16 oz	559	8	89	82	515
Chicken w/ Green Salad	13 oz	377	6	53	128	502
Chili	3 oz	135	3	3	66	300
Chili Tacos	6 oz	314	8	33	66	425
Chili Tacos Dinner	16 oz	579	8	91	66	685
Chips	3 oz	394	17	56	0	30
Combo Burrito	14 oz	598	11	78	124	838
Combo Burrito Dinner	24 oz	863	11	137	124	1098
Enchilada Sauce	1 oz	6	0	2	0	65
Famouse #5	14 oz	583	5	111	20	637
Guacamole	2 oz	201	5	38	0	220
Mex Cheese	1 oz	100	8	0	24	280
Mixed Greens	4 oz	tr	0	0	0	20
Nacho Grande	8 oz	704	38	61	74	625
Rice	6 oz	274	0	64	0	300
Salad w/ Marinated Veggies, Large	8 oz	54	1	11	2	130
Salad w/ Marinated Veggies, Small	5 oz	32	1	6	2	85
Sour Cream Blend	1 oz	27	3	1	8	20
Tortilla, Corn	2 oz	128	0	29	0	10
Tortilla, Flour	2 oz	160	2	32	0	140
Tortilla Mini, Corn	3 oz	160	0	36	0	13
Tortilla, Whole Wheat	2 oz	160	2	30	0	130
Vegetables	4 oz	43	0	11	8	80
Vegetarian Burrito	14 oz	601	7	112	20	748

FOOD	PORTION	CAL	FAT	CARB	CHOL	SOD
Vegetarian Burrito Dinner	24 oz	866	7	170	20	1008
Vegetarian Plate	15 oz	531	5	110	0	429
Vegetarian Tacos	6 oz	295	6	45	22	265
Vegetarian Tacos Dinner	16 oz	560	6	103	22	525
Veggie Taco Salad, Large	17 oz	647	13	112	20	670
Veggie Taco Salad, Small	10 oz	379	8	67	10	425
Yogurt, Nonfat	1 oz	15	0	2	1	22

MCDONALD'S

FAST FACT
The first McDonald's was opened in 1948 in San Bernardino, California. There are now 13,666 worldwide.

FOOD	PORTION	CAL	FAT	CARB	CHOL	SOD
BAKED SELECTIONS						
Apple Danish	1	390	17	51	25	370
Apple Pie	1 (3 oz)	260	15	30	6	240
Chocolaty Chip Cookies	1 pkg (2 oz)	330	15	42	4	280
Cinnamon Raisin Danish	1	440	13	58	34	430
Iced Cheese Danish	1	390	21	42	47	420
McDonaldland Cookies	1 pkg (2 oz)	290	9	47	0	300
Raspberry Danish	1	410	16	62	26	310
BEVERAGES						
Apple Juice	6 oz	90	0	50	0	5
Coca-Cola Classic	16 oz	145	0	40	0	15
Diet Coke	16 fl oz	1	0	tr	0	20
Grapefruit Juice	6 oz	80	0	19	0	0
Milk, 1%	8 oz	110	2	12	10	130

FOOD	PORTION	CAL	FAT	CARB	CHOL	SOD
Milk Shake, Lowfat Chocolate	10.4 oz	320	1	66	10	240
Milk Shake, Lowfat Strawberry	10.4 oz	320	1	67	10	170
Milk Shake, Lowfat Vanilla	10.4 oz	290	1	60	10	170
Orange Drink	16 fl oz	130	0	35	0	15
Orange Juice	6 oz	80	0	19	0	0
Sprite	16 fl oz	145	0	40	0	35
BREAKFAST SELECTIONS						
Biscuit w/ Bacon, Egg & Cheese	1	440	26	33	240	1215
Biscuit w/ Sausage	1	420	28	32	44	1040
Biscuit w/ Sausage & Egg	1	505	33	33	260	1210
Biscuit w/ Spread	1	260	13	32	1	730
Breakfast Burrito	1	280	17	21	135	580
Cheerios	¾ cup	80	1	14	0	210
Egg McMuffin	1	280	11	28	235	710
English Muffin w/ Spread	1	170	4	26	0	285
Fat-Free Apple Bran Muffin	1	180	0	40	0	200
Hash Brown Potatoes	1 serv	130	7	15	0	330
Hotcakes w/ Margarine & Syrup	1 serv	440	12	74	8	685
Sausage	1	160	15	0	43	310
Sausage McMuffin	1	345	20	27	57	770
Sausage McMuffin w/ Egg	1	430	25	27	270	920
Scrambled Eggs	1 serv	140	10	1	425	290
Wheaties	¾ cup	90	1	19	0	220

FOOD	PORTION	CAL	FAT	CARB	CHOL	SOD
ICE CREAM						
Lowfat Frozen Yogurt Sundae w/ Hot Caramel	1 (6 oz)	270	3	59	13	180
Lowfat Frozen Yogurt Sundae w/ Hot Fudge	1 (6 oz)	240	3	50	6	170
Strawberry Lowfat Frozen Yogurt Sundae	1 (6 oz)	210	1	49	5	95
Vanilla Lowfat Frozen Yogurt Cone	1 (3 oz)	105	1	22	3	80
MAIN MENU SELECTIONS						
Big Mac	1	500	26	42	100	890
Cheeseburger	1	305	13	30	50	725
Chicken Fajita	1 (2.9 oz)	190	8	20	35	310
Chicken McNuggets	4 (2.6 oz)	180	10	11	35	390
Chicken McNuggets	6 (3.8 oz)	270	15	17	55	580
Chicken McNuggets	9 (5.6 oz)	405	22	25	85	870
Fillet-O-Fish	1	370	18	38	50	730
French Fries	1 lg serv	400	22	46	0	200
French Fries	1 med serv	320	17	36	0	150
French Fries	1 sm serv	220	12	26	0	110
Hamburger	1	255	9	30	37	490
McChicken	1	415	19	39	50	830
McLean Deluxe	1	320	10	35	60	670
McLean Deluxe w/ Cheese	1	370	14	35	75	890
McNuggets Sauce						
Barbeque	1.12 oz	50	1	12	0	340
Honey	0.5 oz	45	0	12	0	0
Hot Mustard	1.05 oz	70	4	8	5	250
Sweet 'N Sour	1.12 oz	60	tr	14	0	190
Quarter Pounder	1	410	20	34	85	645

FOOD	PORTION	CAL	FAT	CARB	CHOL	SOD
Quarter Pounder w/ Cheese	1	510	28	34	115	1110
SALAD DRESSINGS						
Bleu Cheese	1 pkg	250	20	5	35	750
Lite Vinaigrette	1 pkg	48	2	8	0	240
Ranch	1 pkg	220	20	4	20	520
Red French Reduced Calorie	1 pkg	160	8	20	0	460
Thousand Island	1 pkg	225	20	10	40	500
SALADS AND SALAD BAR						
Bacon Bits	0.1 oz	15	1	0	1	95
Chef Salad	1 serv	170	9	8	111	400
Chunky Chicken Salad	1 serv	150	4	7	78	230
Croutons	0.3 oz	50	2	7	0	140
Garden Salad	1	50	2	6	65	70
Side Salad	1 serv	30	4	4	33	35

MORRISON'S

FOOD	PORTION	CAL	FAT	CARB	CHOL	SOD
DESSERT						
Boston Cream Cake	1 slice	218	4	—	—	171
MAIN MENU SELECTIONS						
Baked Potato	1	220	tr	—	—	16
Broccoli	1 serv (4 oz)	37	2	—	—	310
Cabbage	1 serv (4 oz)	36	tr	—	—	190
Cantaloupe Compote	1 serv (4 oz)	130	1	—	—	30
Cauliflower	1 serv (4 oz)	68	5	—	—	178
Chicken Stew & Dumplings	1 serv (7 oz)	362	14	—	—	468
Chicken Teriyaki	1 serv (5.5 oz)	232	10	—	—	1187
French Bread	1 slice	207	2	—	—	413
Grilled Chicken Pecan Salad	1 serv (6 oz)	298	8	—	—	635
Lima Beans	1 serv (4 oz)	170	4	—	—	300

FOOD	PORTION	CAL	FAT	CARB	CHOL	SOD
Okra & Tomatoes	1 serv (5 oz)	40	2	—	—	233
Pinto Beans	1 serv (4 oz)	105	4	—	—	332
Plain Jell-O	1 serv (3 oz)	131	tr	—	—	109
Rutabagas	1 serv (4 oz)	33	1	—	—	147
Sliced Tomato	4 slices	40	1	—	—	20
Soft Roll	1 (2 oz)	170	4	—	—	200
Strawberries & Bananas Bowl	1 serv (6 oz)	203	1	—	—	4
Strawberries, Peaches & Bananas	1 serv (6 oz)	203	1	—	—	4
Turnip Greens	1 serv (4 oz)	30	2	—	—	365
Watermelon	1 serv (6 oz)	102	1	—	—	6
Yellow Squash	1 serv (4 oz)	22	1	—	—	179
SALADS AND SALAD BAR						
Garden Salad	1 serv (2.5 oz)	75	2	—	—	163
Tossed Salad	1 serv (3 oz)	30	tr	—	—	18

NATHAN'S

FOOD	PORTION	CAL	FAT	CARB	CHOL	SOD
BEVERAGE						
Lemonade	16 fl oz	189	0	46	—	5
Lemonade	22 fl oz	260	0	64	—	7
Lemonade	32 fl oz	378	0	93	—	10
MAIN MENU SELECTIONS						
Breaded Chicken Sandwich	1 (7.2 oz)	510	25	48	56	927
Charbroiled Chicken Sandwich	1 (4.5 oz)	288	5	24	53	861
Cheese Steak Sandwich	1 (6.1 oz)	485	26	37	73	579
Chicken, 2 Pieces	1 serv (7.1 oz)	693	44	26	211	958
Chicken, 4 Pieces	1 serv (14.2 oz)	1382	88	52	422	1912
Chicken Platter, 2 Pieces	1 serv (14.8 oz)	1096	66	72	212	1413

FOOD	PORTION	CAL	FAT	CARB	CHOL	SOD
Chicken Platter, 4 Pieces	1 serv (21.9 oz)	1788	109	99	425	2369
Chicken Salad	1 serv (12.7 oz)	154	4	9	49	345
Double Burger	1 (7.3 oz)	671	41	32	154	460
Fillet of Fish Platter	1 serv (22 oz)	1455	74	137	147	1837
Fillet of Fish Sandwich	1 (5.2 oz)	403	15	46	32	714
Frank Nuggets	15 (6.9 oz)	764	52	54	99	1594
Frank Nuggets	11 (5.1 oz)	563	38	40	73	1173
Frank Nuggets	7 (3.2 oz)	357	24	25	46	744
Frankfurter	1 (3.2 oz)	310	19	22	45	820
French Fries	1 serv (8.6 oz)	514	26	62	0	61
Fried Clam Platter	1 serv (13.1 oz)	1024	51	119	49	1826
Fried Clam Sandwich	1 (5.4 oz)	620	29	72	44	1417
Fried Shrimp	1 serv (4.4 oz)	348	11	47	71	869
Fried Shrimp Platter	1 serv (12.6 oz)	796	34	100	83	1436
Hamburger	1 (4.7 oz)	434	23	32	77	281
Knish	1 (5.9 oz)	318	7	53	2	822
Pastrami Sandwich	1 (4.1 oz)	325	12	34	48	1013
Sautéed Onions	1 serv (3.5 oz)	39	1	6	0	16
Super Burger	1 (7.6 oz)	533	32	34	86	525
Turkey Sandwich	1 (4.9 oz)	270	2	34	27	1458
SALAD AND SALAD BAR						
Garden Salad	1 serv (10.9 oz)	193	13	10	36	261

OLIVE GARDEN

FOOD	PORTION	CAL	FAT	CARB	CHOL	SOD
Baked Lasagna	1 lunch serv	330	18	—	60	1030
Breadstick w/ margarine	1	70	2	—	0	365
Breadstick w/o margarine	1	30	0	—	0	365

FOOD	PORTION	CAL	FAT	CARB	CHOL	SOD
Breadstick w/o margarine or garlic salt	1	30	0	—	0	30
Eggplant Parmigiana	1 lunch serv	220	14	—	45	720
Fettuccine Alfredo	1 lunch serv	790	50	—	160	820
Garden Salad	1 serv	230	15	—	4	560
Minestrone Soup	6 fl oz	45	tr	—	0	220
Pasta & Fagioli	6 fl oz	140	5	—	15	470
Salad Dressing	1 tbsp	60	7	—	2	230
Spaghetti w/ Marinara Sauce	1 lunch serv	315	8	—	tr	768
Spaghetti w/ Tomato Sauce	1 lunch serv	400	9	—	75	1196
Veal Marsala	1 dinner serv	330	29	—	100	460
Veal Parmigiana	1 dinner serv	590	40	—	150	1120
Veal Piccata	1 dinner serv	230	16	—	45	150
Venetian Grilled Chicken w/o pasta or vegetable	1 dinner serv	320	12	—	140	500

PIZZA HUT

FOOD	PORTION	CAL	FAT	CARB	CHOL	SOD
Beef						
Medium Hand Tossed	1 slice	261	10	28	25	795
Medium Pan	1 slice	288	18	27	25	675
Medium Thin 'N Crispy	1 slice	231	11	20	25	705
Cheese						
Big Foot	1 slice	179	5	25	14	959
Medium Hand Tossed	1 slice	253	9	19	25	593
Medium Pan	1 slice	279	13	26	25	473
Medium Thin 'N Crispy	1 slice	223	10	19	25	503

FOOD	PORTION	CAL	FAT	CARB	CHOL	SOD
Chunky Combo						
Hand Tossed	1 slice	280	12	28	29	823
Pan	1 slice	306	16	26	29	703
Thin 'N Crispy	1 slice	250	13	20	29	736
Chunky Meat						
Hand Tossed	1 slice	325	16	28	40	970
Pan	1 slice	352	20	27	40	850
Thin 'N Crispy	1 slice	295	17	20	40	882
Chunky Veggie						
Hand Tossed	1 slice	224	6	29	17	633
Pan	1 slice	251	10	21	17	513
Thin 'N Crispy	1 slice	193	8	28	17	546
Italian Sausage						
Medium Hand Tossed	1 slice	313	15	27	38	871
Medium Pan	1 slice	399	24	28	38	751
Medium Thin 'N Crispy	1 slice	282	17	20	38	781
Meat Lovers						
Medium Hand Tossed	1 slice	321	15	28	42	1106
Medium Pan	1 slice	347	23	27	42	986
Medium Thin 'N Crispy	1 slice	297	16	20	44	1068
Pepperoni						
Big Foot	1 slice	195	7	25	17	1022
Medium Hand Tossed	1 slice	253	10	28	25	738
Medium Pan	1 slice	280	18	26	25	618
Medium Thin 'N Crispy	1 slice	230	11	20	27	678
Personal Pan	1 pie	675	29	76	53	1335
Pepperoni Lovers						
Medium Hand Tossed	1 slice	335	16	28	43	981

FOOD	PORTION	CAL	FAT	CARB	CHOL	SOD
Medium Pan	1 slice	362	25	27	34	861
Medium Thin 'N Crispy	1 slice	320	19	20	46	949
Pepperoni, Italian Sausage & Mushroom, Big Foot	1 slice	213	8	25	21	1208
Pork						
Medium Hand Tossed	1 slice	270	11	28	25	803
Medium Pan	1 slice	296	19	27	25	683
Medium Thin 'N Crispy	1 slice	240	12	20	25	713
Super Supreme						
Medium Hand Tossed	1 slice	276	10	28	32	980
Medium Pan	1 slice	302	19	27	32	860
Medium Thin 'N Crispy	1 slice	253	12	20	35	700
Supreme						
Medium Hand Tossed	1 slice	289	12	28	29	894
Medium Pan	1 slice	315	16	27	29	774
Medium Thin 'N Crispy	1 slice	262	14	20	31	819
Personal Pan	1 pie	647	28	76	53	1313
Veggie Lovers						
Medium Hand Tossed	1 slice	222	7	28	17	641
Medium Pan	1 slice	249	15	27	17	521
Medium Thin 'N Crispy	1 slice	192	8	20	17	551

PONDEROSA

BEVERAGES

Cherry Coke	6 oz	77	0	20	0	4

FOOD	PORTION	CAL	FAT	CARB	CHOL	SOD
Chocolate Milk	8 oz	208	9	26	33	149
Coca-Cola Classic	6 oz	72	0	19	0	7
Coffee, Black	6 oz	2	0	tr	0	26
Diet Coke	6 oz	tr	0	tr	0	8
Diet Coke Caffeine Free	6 oz	tr	0	tr	0	8
Diet Sprite	6 oz	2	0	0	0	4
Dr Pepper	6 oz	72	0	19	0	14
Lemonade	6 oz	68	0	19	0	50
Milk	8 oz	159	9	12	34	122
Mr. Pibb	6 oz	71	0	18	0	10
Orange Soda	6 oz	82	0	21	0	0
Root Beer	6 oz	80	0	21	0	9
Sprite	6 oz	72	0	18	0	16
Tea	6 oz	2	0	1	0	0
ICE CREAM						
Caramel Topping	1 oz	100	1	26	2	72
Chocolate Ice Milk	3.5 oz	152	3	30	22	70
Chocolate Topping	1 oz	89	tr	24	0	37
Strawberry Topping	1 oz	71	tr	24	0	29
Vanilla Ice Milk	3.5 oz	150	3	30	20	58
Whipped Topping	1 oz	80	6	5	0	16
MAIN MENU SELECTIONS						
Baked Beans	1 serv (4 oz)	170	6	21	0	330
Baked Potato	1 (7.2 oz)	145	tr	33	0	6
Bake 'R Broil Fish	1 serv (5.2 oz)	230	13	10	50	330
BBQ Sauce	1 tbsp	25	0	5	0	260
Breaded Cauliflower	1 serv (4 oz)	115	1	23	1	446
Breaded Okra	1 serv (4 oz)	124	1	23	1	483
Breaded Onion Rings	1 serv (4 oz)	213	9	30	2	620
Breaded Zucchini	1 serv (4 oz)	102	1	18	1	584

FOOD	PORTION	CAL	FAT	CARB	CHOL	SOD
Carrots	1 serv (3.5 oz)	31	tr	7	0	33
Cheese Herb Garlic Spread	1 tbsp	100	10	0	0	120
Cheese Sauce	2 oz	52	2	6	4	355
Chicken Breast	1 serv (5.5 oz)	90	2	1	54	400
Chicken Wings	2	213	9	11	75	610
Chopped Steak	5.3 oz	296	22	1	105	296
Chopped Steak	4 oz	225	16	1	80	150
Corn	1 serv (3.5 oz)	90	tr	21	0	5
Fish, Fried	1 serv (3.2 oz)	190	9	17	15	170
Fish Nuggets	1	31	2	2	8	52
French Fries	1 serv (3 oz)	120	4	17	3	39
Gravy, Brown	2 oz	25	1	4	0	167
Gravy, Turkey	2 oz	25	tr	5	0	228
Green Beans	1 serv (3.5 oz)	20	0	3	0	391
Halibut, Broiled	1 serv (6 oz)	170	2	0	—	68
Hot Dog	1	144	13	1	27	460
Italian Breadstick	1	100	1	19	0	200
Kansas City Strip	5 oz	138	6	1	76	850
Macaroni & Cheese	4 oz	67	2	18	4	320
Margarine, Liquid	1 tbsp	100	11	0	0	110
Mashed Potatoes	1 serv (4 oz)	62	tr	13	20	191
Meatballs	1	58	2	1	11	8
Mini Shrimp	6	47	tr	6	22	125
New York Strip, Choice	10 oz	314	15	1	50	1420
New York Strip, Choice	8 oz	384	11	2	62	570
Pasta Shells, Plain	2 oz	78	tr	16	0	tr
Peas	1 serv (3.5 oz)	67	tr	12	0	120
Porterhouse	13 oz	441	30	1	67	1844

FOOD	PORTION	CAL	FAT	CARB	CHOL	SOD
Porterhouse, Choice	16 oz	640	31	3	82	1130
Potato Wedges	1 serv (3.5 oz)	130	6	16	—	171
Rib Eye	5 oz	219	13	1	75	1130
Rib Eye, Choice	6 oz	281	14	tr	60	570
Rice Pilaf	1 serv (4 oz)	160	4	26	22	450
Roll, Dinner	1	184	3	33	0	311
Roll, Sourdough	1	110	1	22	0	230
Roughy, Broiled	1 serv (5 oz)	139	5	—	28	88
Salmon, Broiled	1 serv (6 oz)	192	3	3	60	72
Sandwich Steak	4 oz	408	11	2	62	850
Scrod, Baked	1 serv (7 oz)	120	1	0	65	80
Shrimp, Fried	7	231	tr	31	105	612
Sirloin, Choice	7 oz	241	11	1	63	570
Sirloin Tips, Choice	5 oz	473	8	2	72	280
Spaghetti, Plain	2 oz	78	tr	16	0	tr
Spaghetti Sauce	4 oz	110	4	17	0	520
Steak Kabobs, Meat Only	3 oz	153	5	2	67	280
Stuffing	4 oz	230	11	27	22	800
Sweet & Sour Sauce	1 oz	37	1	8	0	80
Swordfish, Broiled	1 serv (6 oz)	271	9	0	85	0
T-Bone	8 oz	176	9	1	71	850
T-Bone, Choice	10 oz	444	18	2	80	850
Teriyaki Steak	5 oz	174	3	5	64	1420
Tortilla Chips	1 oz	150	8	16	0	80
Trout, Broiled	1 serv (5 oz)	228	4	1	110	51
Winter Mix	1 serv (3.5 oz)	25	0	4	0	33
SALADS AND SALAD BAR						
Alfalfa Sprouts	1 oz	10	0	1	0	0
Apple	1	80	1	20	0	1

FOOD	PORTION	CAL	FAT	CARB	CHOL	SOD
Apples, Canned	4 oz	90	0	22	0	15
Applesauce	4 oz	80	0	20	0	20
Banana	1	87	tr	23	0	1
Banana Chips	0.2 oz	25	1	3	0	tr
Banana Pudding	1 oz	52	2	6	0	29
Bean Sprouts	1 oz	10	tr	2	0	1
Beets, Diced	4 oz	55	tr	13	0	307
Breadsticks, Sesame	2	35	0	6	0	60
Broccoli	1 oz	9	1	2	0	4
Cabbage, Green	1 oz	9	0	2	0	7
Cabbage, Red	1 oz	1	0	tr	0	1
Cantaloupe	1 wedge	13	0	3	0	5
Carrots	1 oz	12	tr	3	0	13
Cauliflower	1 oz	8	tr	2	0	4
Celery	1 oz	4	0	1	0	36
Cheese, Imitation Shredded	1 oz	90	7	1	5	420
Cheese Spread	1 oz	98	7	4	26	188
Cherry Peppers	2 pieces	7	tr	1	0	415
Chicken Salad	3.5 oz	212	15	8	42	335
Chow Mein Noodles	0.2 oz	25	1	3	0	42
Cocktail Sauce	1 oz	34	1	6	0	453
Coconut, Shredded	0.2 oz	25	2	2	0	14
Cottage Cheese	4 oz	120	5	5	17	330
Croutons	1 oz	115	4	18	0	351
Cucumber	1 oz	4	0	1	0	2
Eggs, Diced	2 oz	94	7	1	260	75
Fruit Cocktail	4 oz	97	tr	25	0	7
Garbanzo Beans	1 oz	102	0	17	0	7
Gelatin, Plain	4 oz	71	0	17	0	73

FOOD	PORTION	CAL	FAT	CARB	CHOL	SOD
Granola	0.2 oz	24	1	3	0	—
Grapes	10	34	tr	9	0	2
Ham, Diced	2 oz	120	10	1	76	780
Honeydew	1 wedge	24	tr	6	0	9
Lemon	1 wedge	3	tr	1	0	0
Lettuce	1 oz	5	0	2	0	5
Macaroni Salad	3.5 oz	335	12	49	9	431
Margarine, Whipped	1 tbsp	34	1	0	0	65
Meal Mates Sesame Crackers	2	45	2	6	0	95
Melba Snacks	2	18	0	4	0	60
Mousse, Chocolate	1 oz	78	4	7	0	18
Mousse, Strawberry	1 oz	74	5	6	0	17
Mushrooms	1 oz	8	tr	1	0	4
Olive, Black	1	4	tr	tr	0	24
Olive, Green	1	3	tr	tr	0	69
Onion, Green	1 oz	7	tr	2	0	1
Onions, Red & Yellow	1 oz	11	0	3	3	3
Orange	1	45	tr	11	0	1
Pasta Salad	3.5 oz	269	12	34	tr	441
Peaches, Canned	4 oz	70	0	18	0	10
Peanuts, Chopped	0.2 oz	30	2	1	0	—
Pears, Canned	4 oz	98	tr	25	0	7
Pepper, Green	1 oz	6	tr	1	0	4
Pickles, Dill Spears	0.14 oz	tr	0	tr	0	54
Pickles, Sweet Chips	0.14 oz	4	0	1	0	tr
Pineapple, Fresh	1 wedge	11	tr	3	0	tr
Pineapple Tidbits	4 oz	95	tr	25	0	2
Potato Salad	3.5 oz	126	6	16	7	300
Radishes	1 oz	4	0	1	0	5

FOOD	PORTION	CAL	FAT	CARB	CHOL	SOD
Ritz Crackers	2	40	2	4	0	50
Saltine Crackers	2	25	tr	4	0	38
Spiced Apple Rings	4 oz	100	0	24	0	20
Spinach	1 oz	7	tr	1	0	20
Strawberries	2 oz	14	tr	3	—	61
Strawberry Glaze	1 oz	37	0	10	—	4
Sunflower Seeds	0.2 oz	31	0	1	0	—
Tartar Sauce	1 oz	85	11	11	9	477
Tomatoes	1 oz	6	tr	1	0	1
Turkey Ham Salad	3.5 oz	186	13	10	12	655
Turkey Julienne	1 oz	29	tr	1	15	192
Vanilla Wafers	2	35	1	6	5	25
Watermelon	1 wedge	111	1	27	0	4
Yogurt, Fruit	4 oz	115	1	23	5	70
Yogurt, Vanilla	4 oz	110	2	18	6	75
Zucchini	1 oz	5	0	1	0	tr
SALAD DRESSINGS Blue Cheese	1 oz	130	13	1	27	266
Coleslaw	1 oz	150	14	6	31	284
Creamy Italian	1 oz	103	10	3	0	373
Cucumber Reduced Calorie	1 oz	69	6	3	tr	315
Italian Reduced Calorie	1 oz	31	3	1	0	371
Parmesan Pepper	1 oz	150	15	2	9	282
Ranch	1 oz	147	15	1	3	298
Salad Oil	1 tbsp	120	14	0	0	0
Sour Cream	1 tbsp	26	3	1	5	6
Sweet-N-Tangy	1 oz	122	9	9	1	347
Thousand Island	1 oz	113	10	9	1	405

FOOD	PORTION	CAL	FAT	CARB	CHOL	SOD
POPEYE'S						
Apple Pie	1 serv (3.1 oz)	290	16	37	10	820
Biscuit	1 serv (2.3 oz)	250	15	26	<5	430
Cajun Rice	1 serv (3.9 oz)	150	5	17	25	1260
Chicken Breast, Mild	1 (3.7 oz)	270	16	9	60	660
Chicken Breast, Spicy	1 (3.7 oz)	270	16	9	60	660
Chicken Leg, Mild	1 (1.7 oz)	120	7	4	40	240
Chicken Leg, Spicy	1 (1.7 oz)	120	7	4	40	240
Chicken Thigh, Mild	1 (3.1 oz)	300	23	9	70	620
Chicken Thigh, Spicy	1 (3.1 oz)	300	23	9	70	620
Chicken Wing, Mild	1 (1.6 oz)	160	11	7	40	290
Chicken Wing, Spicy	1 (1.6 oz)	160	11	7	40	290
Coleslaw	1 serv (4 oz)	149	11	14	3	271
Corn on the Cob	1 serv (5.2 oz)	90	3	21	0	20
French Fries	1 serv (3 oz)	240	12	31	10	610
Nuggets	1 serv (4.2 oz)	410	32	18	55	660
Onion Rings	1 serv (3.1 oz)	310	19	31	25	210
Potatoes & Gravy	1 serv w/ 3.8 fl oz	100	6	11	<5	460
Red Beans & Rice	1 serv (5.9 oz)	270	17	30	10	680
Shrimp	1 serv (2.8 oz)	250	16	13	110	650

PUDGIE'S FAMOUS CHICKEN

Fried Chicken	3.5 oz	233	13	4	81	440

QUINCY'S FAMILY STEAKHOUSE

MAIN MENU SELECTIONS

Baked Potato	1 (12 oz)	370	1	86	—	45
Broccoli Spears	1 serv (10 oz)	110	1	14	—	30
Chicken Breast, Grilled	5 oz	120	2	2	—	500

FOOD	PORTION	CAL	FAT	CARB	CHOL	SOD
Filet Mignon	7 oz	330	12	0	—	160
Peppers & Onions	1 serv (4.5 oz)	90	5	10	—	1150
Rainbow Trout, Grilled	6 oz	240	10	0	—	50
Rib Eye	10 oz	670	60	0	—	205
Rib Eye, Thick	13 oz	870	78	0	—	300
Rice Pilaf	1 serv (4 oz)	180	3	35	0	460
Sirloin Club	6 oz	280	10	0	—	160
Sirloin, Large	10 oz	850	70	0	—	240
Sirloin, Petite	5.5 oz	450	37	0	—	120
Sirloin, Regular	8 oz	650	54	0	—	210
Stir-Fry Beef	1 serv (16 oz)	950	77	20	130	590
Stir-Fry Chicken	1 serv (16 oz)	790	67	22	80	1000
T-Bone	14 oz	1610	159	0	—	390
Yeast Roll	1 (1.5 oz)	160	4	29	—	280
SOUP						
Clam Chowder	9 oz	198	14	—	—	—

RAX

FOOD	PORTION	CAL	FAT	CARB	CHOL	SOD
BEVERAGES						
Chocolate Shake	1 (11 fl oz)	445	12	77	35	248
Coca-Cola Classic	16 fl oz	205	0	53	0	11
Diet Coke	16 fl oz	1	0	0	0	21
DESSERT						
Chocolate Chip Cookie	1 (2 oz)	262	12	36	6	192
MAIN MENU SELECTIONS						
Bacon	1 slice (0.1 oz)	14	1	0	2	40
Baked Potato	1 (10 oz)	264	0	61	0	15
Baked Potato w/ 1 tbsp Margarine	1 (10.5 oz)	364	11	61	0	115
Barbecue Sauce	1 pkg (0.4 oz)	11	0	3	0	158

FOOD	PORTION	CAL	FAT	CARB	CHOL	SOD
Beef, Bacon 'N Cheddar	1 (6.7 oz)	523	32	37	42	1042
Cheddar Cheese Sauce	1 oz	29	tr	4	0	225
Country Fried Chicken Breast Sandwich	1 (7.4 oz)	618	29	49	45	1078
Deluxe Roast Beef	1 (7.9 oz)	498	30	39	36	864
French Fries	1 serv (3.25 oz)	282	14	36	3	75
Grilled Chicken Breast Sandwich	1 (6.9 oz)	402	23	26	69	872
Grilled Chicken Garden Salad w/ French Dressing	1 serv (12.7 oz)	477	31	34	32	1189
Grilled Chicken Garden Salad w/ Lite Italian Dressing	1 serv (12.7 oz)	264	12	22	32	1040
Mushroom Sauce	1 oz	16	tr	1	0	113
Philly Melt	1 (8.2 oz)	396	16	40	27	1055
Regular Rax	1 (4.7 oz)	262	10	25	15	707
Swiss Slice	1 slice (0.4 oz)	42	3	0	10	157
SALAD DRESSINGS						
French	2 oz	275	22	20	0	442
Lite Italian	2 oz	63	3	8	0	294
SALADS AND SALAD BAR						
Gourmet Garden w/ French Dressing	1 serv (10.7 oz)	409	29	33	10	792
Gourmet Garden w/ Lite Italian Dressing	1 serv (10.7 oz)	305	10	22	2	643
Gourmet Garden w/o Dressing	1 serv (8.7 oz)	134	6	13	2	350
Grilled Chicken Garden w/o Dressing	1 serv (10.7 oz)	202	9	14	32	747

FOOD	PORTION	CAL	FAT	CARB	CHOL	SOD
RED LOBSTER						
Atlantic Cod	1 lunch serv	100	1	0	70	200
Atlantic Ocean Perch	1 lunch serv	130	4	1	75	190
Blacktip Shark	1 lunch serv	150	1	0	60	90
Calamari, Breaded & Fried	1 lunch serv	360	21	30	140	30
Calico Scallops	1 lunch serv	180	2	8	115	60
Catfish	1 lunch serv	170	10	0	85	50
Chicken Breast, Skinless	4 oz	140	3	0	70	60
Deep Sea Scallops	1 lunch serv	130	2	2	50	260
Filet Mignon	8 oz	350	16	0	140	105
Flounder	1 lunch serv	100	1	1	70	95
Grouper	1 lunch serv	110	1	0	65	70
Haddock	1 lunch serv	110	1	2	85	180
Halibut	1 lunch serv	110	1	1	60	105
Hamburger	5 oz	410	28	0	130	115
King Crab Legs	1 lb	170	2	6	100	900
Langostino	1 lunch serv	120	1	2	210	410
Lemon Sole	1 lunch serv	120	1	1	65	90
Mackerel	1 lunch serv	190	12	1	100	250
Maine Lobster	18 oz	240	8	5	310	550
Mako Shark	1 lunch serv	140	1	0	100	60
Monkfish	1 lunch serv	110	1	24	80	95
Norwegian Salmon	1 lunch serv	230	12	3	80	60
Pollack	1 lunch serv	120	1	1	90	90
Rainbow Trout	1 lunch serv	170	9	0	90	90
Red Rockfish	1 lunch serv	90	1	0	85	95
Red Snapper	1 lunch serv	110	1	0	70	140
Rib Eye Steak	12 oz	980	82	0	220	150

FOOD	PORTION	CAL	FAT	CARB	CHOL	SOD
Rock Lobster	1 tail (13 oz)	230	3	2	200	1090
Shrimp	8–12 (7 oz)	120	2	0	230	110
Sirloin Steak	8 oz	350	15	0	150	110
Snow Crab Legs	1 lb	150	2	1	130	1630
Sockeye Salmon	1 lunch serv	160	4	3	50	60
Strip Steak	9 oz	560	40	0	150	115
Swordfish	1 lunch serv	100	4	0	100	140
Tilefish	1 lunch serv	100	2	0	80	60
Yellowfin Tuna	1 lunch serv	180	6	0	70	70

ROY ROGERS

BEVERAGE

Orange Juice	11 fl oz	140	tr	34	0	5

BREAKFAST SELECTIONS

Bagel, Cinnamon Raisin	1 (4 oz)	300	1	63	0	490
Bagel, Plain	1 (4 oz)	300	2	60	0	520
Big Country Platter w/ Bacon	1 serv (7.6 oz)	740	43	61	305	1800
Big Country Platter w/ Ham	1 serv (9.4 oz)	710	39	67	330	2210
Big Country Platter w/ Sausage	1 serv (9.6 oz)	920	60	61	340	2230
Biscuit	1 (2.9 oz)	390	21	44	0	1000
Biscuit						
Bacon	1 (3.1 oz)	420	23	44	5	1140
Bacon & Egg	1 (4.2 oz)	470	26	44	150	1190
Cinnamon 'N' Raisin	1 (2.8 oz)	370	18	48	0	450
Ham & Cheese	1 (4.5 oz)	450	24	48	25	1570
Ham & Egg	1 (5.1 oz)	460	23	48	165	1395
Ham, Egg & Cheese	1 (5.6 oz)	500	27	48	170	1620

FOOD	PORTION	CAL	FAT	CARB	CHOL	SOD
Sausage	1 (4.1 oz)	510	31	44	25	1360
Sausage & Egg	1 (5.2 oz)	560	35	44	170	1400
Hashrounds	1 serv (2.8 oz)	230	14	24	0	560
3 Pancakes	1 serv (4.8 oz)	280	2	56	15	890
3 Pancakes w/ 1 Sausage	1 serv (6.2 oz)	430	16	56	40	1290
3 Pancakes w/ 2 Bacon Strips	1 serv (5.3 oz)	350	9	56	25	1130
Sourdough Ham, Egg & Cheese	1 (6.8 oz)	480	24	45	185	1440
DESSERT Strawberry Shortcake	1 serv (6.6 oz)	480	21	39	40	330
ICE CREAM Hot Fudge Sundae	1 (6 oz)	320	10	50	25	260
Ice Cream Cone	1 (4.1 oz)	180	4	29	15	80
Strawberry Sundae	1 (5.5 oz)	260	6	44	15	95
MAIN MENU SELECTIONS Bacon Cheeseburger	1 (5.9 oz)	520	31	32	—	740
Baked Beans	1 serv (5 oz)	160	2	30	10	560
Baked Potato	1 (3.9 oz)	130	1	27	0	65
Baked Potato w/ Margarine	1 (4.4 oz)	240	13	27	0	220
Baked Potato w/ Margarine & Sour Cream	1 (5.4 oz)	300	19	28	15	230
Cheeseburger	1 (4.2 oz)	300	13	34	25	690
Chicken Fillet Sandwich	1 (8.3 oz)	500	24	49	20	1050
Coleslaw	1 serv (5 oz)	295	25	16	15	430
Cornbread	1 serv (2.7 oz)	310	17	35	30	260
Fisherman's Fillet	1 (6.5 oz)	490	21	56	15	1040
Fried Chicken Breast	1 (5.2 oz)	370	15	29	75	1190
Fried Chicken Leg	1 (2.4 oz)	170	7	15	45	570

FOOD	PORTION	CAL	FAT	CARB	CHOL	SOD
Fried Chicken Thigh	1 (4.2 oz)	330	15	30	60	1000
Fried Chicken Wing	1 (2.3 oz)	200	8	23	30	740
Fries	1 lg serv (6.1 oz)	430	18	59	0	190
Fries	1 reg serv (5 oz)	350	15	49	0	150
Gravy	1 serv (1.5 oz)	20	tr	3	0	260
Grilled Chicken Sandwich	1 (8.3 oz)	340	11	32	30	910
Hamburger	1 (3.8 oz)	260	9	33	20	460
Mashed Potatoes	1 serv (5 oz)	92	tr	20	0	320
Nuggets	9 (6.2 oz)	460	29	32	25	970
Nuggets	6 (4 oz)	290	18	20	15	610
Pizza	1 serv (4.75 oz)	282	6	44	14	549
Quarter-Pound Cheeseburger	1 (6 oz)	510	26	44	—	620
Quarter-Pound Hamburger	1 (5.5 oz)	460	22	44	—	390
Quarter Roaster Dark Meat	7.4 oz	490	34	2	225	1120
Quarter Roaster Dark Meat, Skinless	4 oz	190	10	1	110	400
Quarter Roaster White Meat	8.6 oz	500	29	3	240	1450
Quarter Roaster White Meat, Skinless	4.7 oz	190	6	2	100	700
Roast Beef Sandwich	1 (5.7 oz)	260	4	30	60	700
Sourdough Grilled Chicken	1 (10.1 oz)	500	21	46	45	1530
Sourdough Bacon Cheeseburger	1 (9.1 oz)	770	50	45	—	1410
SALADS AND SALAD BAR						
Garden Salad	1 (9.3 oz)	190	14	3	40	280
Grilled Chicken Salad	1 serv (9.8 oz)	120	4	2	60	520
Side Salad	1 (4.9 oz)	20	tr	3	0	20

FOOD	PORTION	CAL	FAT	CARB	CHOL	SOD
SCHLOTZSKY'S DELI						
SANDWICHES						
Chicken Breast	1 sm	514	22	—	—	—
Dijon Chicken Breast	1 sm	469	16	—	—	—
The Original	1 sm	598	33	—	—	—
Smoked Turkey	1 sm	510	22	—	—	—
PIZZAS						
Chicken & Pesto	1 serv	634	18	—	—	—
Onion & Mushroom	1 serv	577	20	—	—	—
Smoked Turkey & Jalapeno	1 serv	589	13	—	—	—
Vegetarian	1 serv	555	17	—	—	—
SOUPS						
Creole	1 serv	120	3	—	—	—
Red Bean	1 serv (8 fl oz)	110	2	—	—	—
Shrimp & Okra	1 serv (8 fl oz)	100	3	—	—	—
Spicy Chicken	1 serv (8 fl oz)	120	3	—	—	—
SALADS						
Chicken Chef	1 serv	192	8	—	—	—
Turkey Club	1 serv	233	10	—	—	—
SHAKEY'S						
MAIN MENU SELECTIONS						
3-Piece Fried Chicken & Potatoes	1 serv	947	56	51	—	2293
5-Piece Fried Chicken & Potatoes	1 serv	1700	90	97	—	5327
Hot Ham & Cheese	1	550	21	56	—	2135
Potatoes	15 pieces	950	36	120	—	3703
Spaghetti w/ Meat Sauce & Garlic Bread	1 serv	940	33	134	—	1904
Super Hot Hero	1	810	44	67	—	2688

FOOD	PORTION	CAL	FAT	CARB	CHOL	SOD
PIZZA						
Homestyle Crust Cheese	1 slice	303	14	31	21	591
Homestyle Crust Onion, Green Pepper, Black Olives, Mushrooms	1 slice	320	15	32	21	652
Pepperoni	1 slice	343	15	31	27	740
Sausage, Mushroom	1 slice	343	17	31	24	677
Sausage, Pepperoni	1 slice	374	20	32	24	676
Shakey's Special	1 slice	384	21	32	29	878
Thick Crust Cheese	1 slice	170	5	22	13	421
Green Pepper, Black Olives, Mushrooms	1 slice	162	4	22	13	418
Pepperoni	1 slice	185	6	22	17	422
Sausage, Mushrooms	1 slice	179	6	22	15	420
Sausage, Pepperoni	1 slice	177	8	22	19	424
Shakey's Special	1 slice	208	8	22	18	423
Thin Crust Cheese	1 slice	133	5	13	14	323
Onion, Green Pepper, Black Olives, Mushrooms	1 slice	125	5	14	11	313
Pepperoni	1 slice	148	7	13	14	403
Sausage, Mushroom	1 slice	141	6	13	13	336
Sausage, Pepperoni	1 slice	166	8	13	17	397
Shakey's Special	1 slice	171	9	14	16	475

FOOD	PORTION	CAL	FAT	CARB	CHOL	SOD
SHONEY'S						
BEVERAGES						
Clear Soda	1 lg	105	0	28	0	21
Clear Soda	1 sm	52	0	14	0	10
Coffee, Regular & Decaf	1 cup	8	0	1	0	8
Cola	1 lg	139	0	33	0	10
Cola	1 sm	69	0	17	0	5
Creamer	0.38 oz	14	1	1	0	8
Hot Chocolate	1 cup	110	2	20	154	154
Hot Tea	1 cup	0	0	tr	0	19
Milk, 2%	1 cup	121	5	12	18	122
Orange Juice	4 oz	54	tr	13	0	1
Sugar	1 pkg	13	0	3	0	0
BREAKFAST SELECTIONS						
Ambrosia Salad	¼ cup	75	3	12	0	167
Apple	1	81	1	21	0	1
Apple Butter	1 tbsp	37	tr	9	0	0
Apple Grape Surprise	¼ cup	19	0	5	0	2
Apple Ring	1	15	0	4	0	0
Apple, Sliced	1 slice	13	tr	3	0	0
Bacon	1 strip	36	3	0	5	101
Beef Stick	1	43	1	5	—	17
Biscuit	1	170	8	22	0	364
Blueberries	¼ cup	21	tr	5	0	2
Blueberry Muffin	1	107	4	18	17	1
Bread Pudding	1 sq	305	11	44	80	409
Breakfast Ham	1 slice	26	1	tr	14	263
Brunch Cake						
Apple	1 sq	160	8	19	0	150
Banana	1 sq	152	7	21	0	120

FOOD	PORTION	CAL	FAT	CARB	CHOL	SOD
Brunch Cake *(cont.)*						
Carrot	1 sq	150	7	20	0	159
Pineapple	1 sq	147	7	20	0	120
Sour Cream	1 sq	160	8	21	0	135
Buttered Toast	2 slices	163	5	25	0	296
Cantaloupe, Diced	½ cup	28	tr	7	0	7
Cantaloupe, Sliced	1 slice	8	tr	2	0	2
Captain Crunch Berry	½ cup	73	2	14	0	122
Cheese Sauce	1 ladle	26	2	4	0	166
Chicken Pieces	1 piece	40	2	2	—	28
Chocolate Pudding	¼ cup	81	2	16	7	81
Cinnamon Honey Bun	1	344	12	54	0	169
Cottage Cheese	1 tbsp	12	tr	1	1	66
Cottage Fries	¼ cup	62	2	10	0	124
Country Gravy	¼ cup	82	7	4	1	255
Croissant	1	260	16	22	2	260
Donut, Mini Cinnamon	1	56	3	7	0	65
DoughNugget	1	157	10	15	0	194
Egg, Fried	1	159	15	1	274	69
Egg, Scrambled	¼ cup	95	7	1	248	155
English Muffin w/ Margarine	1	140	2	18	0	1
Fluff	¼ cup	16	0	3	0	0
French Toast	1 slice	69	3	9	0	157
Fruit Delight	¼ cup	54	2	10	0	2
Fruit Topping, All Flavors	1 tbsp	24	0	6	0	3
Glacéed Fruit	¼ cup	51	tr	13	0	5
Golden Pound Cake	1 slice	134	5	20	13	144
Grape Jelly	1 tbsp	60	0	16	0	0

FOOD	PORTION	CAL	FAT	CARB	CHOL	SOD
Grapefruit, Canned	¼ cup	24	tr	6	0	5
Grapes	25	57	1	14	0	2
Grits	¼ cup	57	3	6	0	62
Hash Browns	¼ cup	43	2	7	0	24
Home Fries	¼ cup	53	2	9	0	24
Honey Bun	1	265	14	32	3	33
Honeydew, Sliced	1 slice	13	0	3	0	4
Jelly Packet	1	40	0	10	0	2
Jr. Bun, Chocolate	1	141	5	22	0	70
Jr. Bun, Honey	1	141	5	22	0	70
Jr. Bun, Maple	1	141	5	22	0	70
Kiwi, Sliced	1 slice	11	tr	3	0	1
Marble Cake w/ Icing	1 slice	136	5	22	0	149
Mixed Fruit	¼ cup	37	tr	9	0	3
Mushroom Topping	1 oz	25	2	1	0	323
Oleo, Whipped	1 tbsp	70	8	0	0	97
Omelette Topping	1 spoonful	23	2	1	3	99
100% Natural	½ cup	244	11	33	0	45
Orange	1 med	65	tr	16	0	2
Orange Sections	1 section	7	0	2	0	0
Oriental Salad	¼ cup	79	3	13	1	32
Pancake	1	41	tr	9	0	238
Pear	1	98	1	25	0	1
Pineapple Bits	1 tbsp	9	0	2	0	2
Pineapple, Fresh, Sliced	1 slice	10	tr	3	0	0
Pistachio Pineapple Salad	¼ cup	98	0	20	3	39
Prunes	1 tbsp	19	0	5	0	0
Raisin Bran	½ cup	87	1	22	0	185

FOOD	PORTION	CAL	FAT	CARB	CHOL	SOD
Raisin English Muffin w/ Margarine	1	158	4	27	0	280
Sausage Link	1	91	9	tr	13	291
Sausage Patty	1	136	13	1	2	48
Sausage Rice	¼ cup	110	6	10	8	211
Shortcake	1	60	2	13	0	90
Sirloin Steak, Charbroiled	6 oz	357	25	0	99	160
Smoked Sausage	1	103	10	1	13	39
Snow Salad	¼ cup	72	4	9	0	18
Strawberries	5	23	tr	5	0	1
Syrup, Light	1 ladle	60	0	15	0	0
Syrup, Low-Cal	2.2 oz	98	0	24	0	0
Tangerine	1	37	tr	9	0	1
Trix	½ cup	54	tr	13	0	89
Waldorf Salad	¼ cup	81	5	9	2	68
Watermelon, Diced	½ cup	50	1	12	0	3
Watermelon, Sliced	1 slice	9	tr	2	0	1
Whipped Topping	1 scoop	10	1	1	0	3
CHILDREN'S MENU SELECTIONS						
All-American Jr. Burger	1 serv	234	11	20	30	543
Kid's Chicken Dinner, Fried	1 serv	244	13	11	40	151
Kid's Fish N' Chips w/ Fries	1 serv	337	17	33	41	467
Kid's Fried Shrimp	1 serv	194	12	12	70	633
Kid's Spaghetti	1 serv	247	8	32	27	193
DESSERTS						
Apple Pie A La Mode	1 slice	492	23	67	35	574
Carrot Cake	1 slice	500	26	56	37	476
Strawberry Pie	1 slice	332	17	45	0	247

FOOD	PORTION	CAL	FAT	CARB	CHOL	SOD
Walnut Brownie A La Mode	1	576	34	61	35	435
ICE CREAM						
Hot Fudge Cake	1 slice	522	20	82	27	485
Hot Fudge Sundae	1	451	22	60	60	226
Strawberry Sundae	1	380	19	48	69	145
MAIN MENU SELECTIONS						
All-American Burger	1	501	33	27	86	597
BBQ Sauce	1 serv	41	1	8	0	232
Bacon Burger	1	591	40	29	86	801
Baked Fish	1 serv	170	1	2	83	1641
Baked Fish, Light	1 serv	170	1	2	83	1641
Baked Ham Sandwich	1	290	10	28	42	1263
Baked Potato	10 oz	264	tr	61	0	16
Beef Patty, Light	1 serv	289	23	0	82	187
Charbroiled Chicken	1 serv	239	7	1	85	592
Charbroiled Chicken Sandwich	1	451	17	28	90	1002
Chicken Fillet Sandwich	1	464	21	39	51	585
Chicken Tenders	1 serv	388	20	17	64	239
Cocktail Sauce	1 serv	36	tr	9	0	260
Country Fried Sandwich	1	588	26	67	29	1501
Country Fried Steak	1 serv	449	27	34	27	1177
Fish N' Chips w/ Fries	1 serv	639	35	50	103	873
Fish N' Shrimp	1 serv	487	26	37	127	644
Fish Sandwich	1	323	13	41	21	740
French Fries	4 oz	252	10	39	0	364
Fried Fish, Light	1 serv	297	14	22	65	536
Grecian Bread	1 slice	80	2	13	0	94

FOOD	PORTION	CAL	FAT	CARB	CHOL	SOD
Grilled Bacon & Cheese Sandwich	1	440	28	28	36	1200
Grilled Cheese Sandwich	1	302	17	25	36	880
Half O'Pound	1 serv	435	34	0	123	280
Ham Club on Whole Wheat	1	642	36	45	78	2105
Hawaiian Chicken	1 serv	262	7	7	85	593
Italian Feast	1 serv	500	20	44	74	369
Lasagna	1 serv	297	10	45	26	870
Liver N' Onions	1 serv	411	23	23	529	321
Mushroom Swiss Burger	1	616	42	29	106	1135
Old-Fashioned Burger	1	470	28	26	82	681
Onion Rings	1	52	3	5	2	102
Patty Melt	1	640	42	30	171	826
Philly Steak Sandwich	1	673	44	37	103	1242
Reuben Sandwich	1	596	35	32	138	3873
Rib Eye	6 oz	605	51	0	141	141
Rice	3.5 oz	137	4	23	1	765
Sautéed Mushrooms	3 oz	75	7	4	0	968
Sautéed Onions	2.5 oz	37	2	4	0	221
Seafood Platter	1 serv	566	28	46	127	893
Shoney Burger	1	498	36	22	79	782
Shrimp, Bite-Size	1 serv	387	25	25	140	1266
Shrimp, Broiled	1 serv	93	18	0	182	210
Shrimp, Charbroiled	1 serv	138	3	3	162	170
Shrimp Sampler	1 serv	412	23	26	217	783
Shrimper's Feast	1 serv	383	22	30	125	216
Shrimper's Feast, Large	1 serv	575	33	45	188	324

FOOD	PORTION	CAL	FAT	CARB	CHOL	SOD
Sirloin	6 oz	357	25	0	99	160
Slim Jim Sandwich	1	484	24	40	57	1620
Spaghetti	1 serv	496	16	63	55	387
Steak N' Shrimp (Charbroiled Shrimp)	1 serv	361	23	1	141	198
Steak N' Shrimp (Fried Shrimp)	1 serv	507	33	15	150	249
Sweet N' Sour Sauce	1 serv	58	0	15	0	5
Tartar Sauce	1 serv	84	8	4	11	177
Turkey Club on Whole Wheat	1	635	33	44	100	1289
SALAD DRESSINGS						
Biscayne Lo-Cal	2 tbsp	62	1	1	0	334
Blue Cheese	2 tbsp	113	13	0	15	109
Creamy Italian	2 tbsp	135	15	1	0	454
French	2 tbsp	124	12	2	12	204
Golden Italian	2 tbsp	141	15	1	0	302
Honey Mustard	2 tbsp	165	17	2	18	5
Ranch	2 tbsp	95	10	0	15	10
Rue French	2 tbsp	122	10	2	0	364
Thousand Island	2 tbsp	130	13	2	12	179
Weight Watchers Italian	2 tbsp	10	0	2	0	615
SALADS AND SALAD BAR						
Ambrosia Salad	¼ cup	75	3	12	0	167
Apple Grape Surprise	¼ cup	19	0	5	0	2
Apple Ring	1	15	0	4	0	3
Bacon Bits	1 spoonful	15	1	1	—	—
Beet Onion Salad	¼ cup	25	1	3	0	167
Broccoli	¼ cup	4	tr	1	0	4
Broccoli & Cauliflower	¼ cup	98	9	4	0	478
Broccoli & Cauliflower Ranch Salad	¼ cup	65	6	2	9	12

FOOD	PORTION	CAL	FAT	CARB	CHOL	SOD
Broccoli, Cauliflower, Carrot Salad	¼ cup	53	4	3	1	193
Carrot	¼ cup	10	tr	2	0	8
Carrot Apple Salad	¼ cup	99	9	4	8	10
Cauliflower	¼ cup	8	tr	2	0	5
Celery	1 tbsp	5	0	tr	0	7
Cheese, Shredded	1 tbsp	21	2	tr	2	112
Chocolate Pudding	¼ cup	81	2	16	7	81
Chow Mein Noodles	1 spoonful	13	1	tr	0	0
Coleslaw	¼ cup	69	5	5	7	106
Cottage Cheese	1 tbsp	12	tr	1	1	66
Croutons	1 spoonful	13	tr	2	0	38
Cucumber	1 tbsp	1	0	tr	0	0
Cucumber, Lite	¼ cup	12	tr	3	0	344
Don's Pasta Salad	¼ cup	82	5	9	0	223
Egg, Diced	1 tbsp	15	1	tr	54	14
Fruit Delight	¼ cup	54	2	10	0	2
Fruit Topping, All Flavors	¼ cup	64	tr	16	0	8
Glacéed Fruit	¼ cup	51	tr	13	0	5
Granola	1 spoonful	25	1	3	0	—
Grapefruit	¼ cup	24	tr	6	0	5
Green Pepper	1 tbsp	1	0	tr	0	0
Italian Vegetable Salad	¼ cup	11	tr	3	0	110
Jell-O	¼ cup	40	0	9	0	26
Jell-O Fluff	¼ cup	16	tr	3	0	0
Kidney Bean Salad	¼ cup	55	2	7	2	154
Lettuce	1.8 oz	7	tr	1	0	5
Macaroni Salad	¼ cup	207	14	17	14	382
Margarine, Whipped	1 tsp	23	3	0	0	32

FOOD	PORTION	CAL	FAT	CARB	CHOL	SOD
Melba Toast	2	20	0	4	0	45
Mixed Fruit Salad	¼ cup	37	tr	9	0	3
Mixed Squash	¼ cup	49	4	2	0	230
Mushrooms	1 tbsp	1	0	tr	0	0
Oil	1 tsp	45	5	0	0	0
Olives, Black	2	10	1	0	0	38
Olives, Green	2	8	1	0	0	162
Onion, Sliced	1 tbsp	1	0	tr	0	0
Oriental Salad	¼ cup	79	3	13	1	31
Pea Salad	¼ cup	73	6	4	42	89
Pepperoni	1 tbsp	30	3	0	—	81
Pickle Chip	1	5	0	1	0	30
Pickle Spear	1	2	0	tr	0	271
Pineapple Bits	1 tbsp	9	0	2	0	2
Pistachio Pineapple Salad	¼ cup	98	3	20	0	39
Prunes	1 tbsp	19	0	5	0	0
Radish	1 tbsp	1	0	tr	0	1
Raisins	1 spoonful	26	0	7	0	1
Rotelli Pasta	¼ cup	78	4	9	0	82
Seign Salad	¼ cup	72	4	8	5	122
Snow Delight	¼ cup	72	4	9	0	18
Spaghetti Salad	¼ cup	81	5	9	0	20
Spinach	¼ cup	1	0	tr	0	4
Spring Pasta	¼ cup	38	3	2	0	162
Summer Salad	¼ cup	114	12	2	0	233
Sunflower Seeds	1 spoonful	40	3	1	0	2
Three-Bean Salad	¼ cup	96	5	12	0	189
Trail Mix	1 spoonful	30	0	4	0	0
Turkey Ham	1 tbsp	12	1	tr	1	121

FOOD	PORTION	CAL	FAT	CARB	CHOL	SOD
Waldorf Salad	¼ cup	81	5	9	2	68
Wheat Bread	1 slice	71	1	14	0	150
SOUPS						
Bean	6 fl oz	63	1	10	4	479
Beef Cabbage	6 fl oz	86	3	9	13	503
Broccoli Cauliflower	6 fl oz	124	9	12	12	560
Cheddar Chowder	6 fl oz	91	2	14	—	948
Cheese Florentine Ham	6 fl oz	110	8	12	11	890
Chicken Gumbo	6 fl oz	60	2	7	—	1050
Chicken Noodle	6 fl oz	62	1	9	14	127
Chicken Rice	6 fl oz	72	1	13	6	117
Clam Chowder	6 fl oz	94	5	10	0	66
Corn Chowder	6 fl oz	148	5	22	—	510
Cream of Broccoli	6 fl oz	75	5	11	1	415
Cream of Chicken	6 fl oz	136	9	14	11	1164
Cream of Chicken Vegetable	6 fl oz	79	1	13	—	714
Onion	6 fl oz	29	2	2	1	88
Potato	6 fl oz	102	3	17	0	335
Tomato Florentine	6 fl oz	63	1	11	0	683
Tomato Vegetable	6 fl oz	46	tr	10	0	314
Vegetable Beef	6 fl oz	82	2	14	5	1254

SKIPPER'S

FOOD	PORTION	CAL	FAT	CARB	CHOL	SOD
BEVERAGES						
Coca-Cola Classic	1 (12 fl oz)	144	0	38	0	14
Diet Coke	1 (12 fl oz)	2	0	0	0	8
Lowfat Milk	1 (12 fl oz)	181	10	32	0	225
Root Beer	1 (12 fl oz)	154	0	42	0	31
Root Beer Float	1 (12 oz)	302	10	33	10	66

FOOD	PORTION	CAL	FAT	CARB	CHOL	SOD
Sprite	1 (12 fl oz)	142	0	36	0	45
DESSERT						
Jell-O	1 serv (2.75 oz)	55	0	12	0	35
MAIN MENU SELECTIONS						
Baked Fish w/ Margarine & Seasoning	1 serv (4.4 oz)	147	3	0	85	475
Baked Potato	1 (6 oz)	145	0	32	0	6
Captain's Cut	1 piece (2.6 oz)	160	7	14	29	353
Cocktail Sauce	1 tbsp	20	0	5	0	216
Coleslaw	1 serv (5 oz)	289	27	10	50	329
Corn Muffin	1 (2 oz)	91	5	14	16	135
English Style Fish	1 piece (2.4 oz)	187	12	11	—	415
French Fries	1 serv (3.5 oz)	239	12	29	3	57
Green Salad w/o Dressing	1 serv (4 oz)	24	0	4	0	8
Ketchup	1 tbsp	17	0	4	0	213
Margarine	1 serv (0.5 oz)	50	6	0	0	60
Shrimp, Fried Cajun	1 serv (4 oz)	342	21	27	64	147
Shrimp, Fried Jumbo	1 piece (.65 oz)	51	2	5	9	102
Shrimp, Fried Original	1 serv (4 oz)	266	13	25	54	1089
Tartar, Original	1 tbsp	65	7	0	4	102
SOUP						
Clam Chowder	1 pint (12 fl oz)	200	7	19	24	1050
Clam Chowder	1 cup (6 fl oz)	100	4	14	12	525

SONIC DRIVE-IN

FOOD	PORTION	CAL	FAT	CARB	CHOL	SOD
Bacon Cheeseburger	1 (7.2 oz)	548	39	23	87	839
BLT Sandwich	1 (6.1 oz)	327	19	27	9	600
Breaded Chicken Sandwich	1 (7.4 oz)	455	25	36	42	755
Breaded Steak Sandwich	1 (3.9 oz)	631	42	46	50	1047

FOOD	PORTION	CAL	FAT	CARB	CHOL	SOD
Cheese Coney Extra-Long	1 (8.9 oz)	635	39	45	65	632
Extra-Long w/ Onions	1 (9.4 oz)	640	39	47	65	632
Regular	1 (5 oz)	358	15	23	40	341
Regular w/ Onions	1 (5.3 oz)	361	23	24	40	341
Chili Pie	1 (3.7 oz)	327	23	20	28	313
Corn Dog	1 (3 oz)	280	15	30	35	700
Fish Sandwich	1 (6.1 oz)	277	7	38	6	655
French Fries	1 lg serv (6.7 oz)	315	11	50	11	67
French Fries	1 reg serv (5 oz)	233	8	37	8	50
French Fries w/ Cheese	1 lg serv (7.7 oz)	219	20	51	38	468
Grilled Cheese Sandwich	1 (2.8 oz)	288	17	25	36	841
Grilled Chicken Sandwich w/o Dressing	1 (6.4 oz)	215	4	23	4	716
#1 Hamburger	1 (6.6 oz)	409	27	23	58	444
#2 Hamburger	1 (6.6 oz)	323	16	23	50	549
Hickory Burger	1 (5.1 oz)	314	16	23	50	459
Hot Dog, Regular	1 (3.5 oz)	258	15	21	23	241
Jalapeno Burger, Double Meat & Cheese	1 (9.1 oz)	638	41	22	136	1358
Mini Burger	1 (3.5 oz)	246	11	20	36	510
Mini Cheeseburger	1 (3.9 oz)	281	14	20	45	644
Onion Rings	1 lg serv (5 oz)	577	38	54	—	532
Onion Rings	1 reg serv (3.5 oz)	404	27	38	—	372
Super Sonic Burger w/ Mayo, Double Meat & Cheese	1 (10.1 oz)	730	52	24	144	1023

## TACO BELL 95

FOOD	PORTION	CAL	FAT	CARB	CHOL	SOD
Super Sonic Burger w/ Mustard, Double Meat & Cheese	1 (10.1 oz)	644	41	24	136	1128
Tater Tots	1 serv (3 oz)	150	7	19	10	330
Tater Tots w/ Cheese	1 serv (3.6 oz)	220	13	19	28	569

SUBWAY

FOOD	PORTION	CAL	FAT	CARB	CHOL	SOD
Ham Sandwich Round	1 (4 in)	317	3	—	13	670
Roast Beef Sandwich Round	1 (4 in)	326	2	—	17	820
Roast Turkey Breast Salad	1 serv	154	7	—	31	950
Roast Turkey Breast Sub w/ White Bread	1 (6 in)	312	8	—	31	1190
Subway Club Salad	1 serv	165	7	—	38	1160
Veggies & Cheese Sub w/ Wheat Bread	1 (6 in)	258	6	—	10	530

TACO BELL

FOOD	PORTION	CAL	FAT	CARB	CHOL	SOD
Burrito, Bean	1	381	14	63	9	1148
Burrito, Beef	1	431	21	48	57	1311
Burrito, Chicken	1	334	12	38	52	880
Burrito, Combo	1	407	16	46	33	1136
Burrito Supreme	1	440	22	55	33	1181
Chilito	1	383	18	36	47	893
Cinnamon Twists	1 serv	171	8	24	0	234
Green Sauce	1 oz	4	0	1	0	136
Guacamole	0.6 oz	34	2	3	0	113
Jalapeno Peppers	3.5 oz	20	0	4	0	1370
Mexican Pizza	1	575	37	40	52	1031
MexiMelt, Beef	1	266	15	19	38	689
MexiMelt, Chicken	1	257	15	19	48	779
Nacho Cheese Sauce	2 oz	103	8	5	9	393

FOOD	PORTION	CAL	FAT	CARB	CHOL	SOD
Nachos	1 serv	346	18	37	9	399
Nachos Bellgrande	1	649	35	61	36	997
Nachos Supreme	1	367	27	41	18	471
Pico De Gallo	1 oz	6	0	1	1	88
Pintos 'N Cheese	1	190	9	19	16	642
Ranch Dressing	2.5 oz	236	25	1	35	571
Red Sauce	1 oz	10	0	2	0	261
Salsa	0.3 oz	18	0	4	0	376
Sour Cream	0.66 oz	46	4	1	0	0
Taco	1	183	11	11	32	276
Taco Salad	1	905	61	55	80	910
Taco Salad w/o Shell	1	484	31	22	80	680
Taco Sauce	1 pkg	2	0	0	0	126
Taco Sauce, Hot	1 pkg	3	0	0	0	82
Taco, Soft	1	225	12	18	32	554
Taco, Soft, Chicken	1	213	10	19	52	615
Taco, Soft, Supreme	1	272	16	19	32	554
Taco Supreme	1	230	15	12	32	276
Tostada	1	243	11	27	16	596

TACO JOHN'S

FOOD	PORTION	CAL	FAT	CARB	CHOL	SOD
Bean Burrito	1	197	6	37	—	636
Beef Burrito	1	303	18	25	—	666
Chicken Burrito w/ Green Chili	1	344	16	29	—	986
Chicken Super Taco Salad w/ Dressing	1	507	27	61	—	1232
Chicken Super Taco Salad w/o Dressing	1	377	15	56	—	882
Chimichanga	1	464	21	67	—	1246
Chimichanga w/ Chicken	1	441	19	55	—	1234

FOOD	PORTION	CAL	FAT	CARB	CHOL	SOD
Combo Burrito	1	250	12	31	—	651
Mexican Rice	1 serv	340	8	59	—	1280
Nachos	1 serv	468	25	45	—	444
Potato Ole	1 lg	414	6	96	—	1595
Smothered Burrito w/ Green Chili	1	367	18	18	—	998
Smothered Burrito w/ Texas Chili	1	455	23	47	—	1217
Softshell	1	224	13	23	—	506
Softshell w/ Chicken	1	180	8	20	—	490
Super Burrito	1	389	16	51	—	856
Super Burrito w/ Chicken	1	366	14	40	—	844
Super Nachos	1 serv	669	39	60	—	994
Super Taco Bravo	1	361	19	43	—	826
Super Taco Salad w/ 2 oz Dressing	1	558	32	65	—	1250
Super Taco Salad w/o Dressing	1	428	20	59	—	900
Taco	1	178	13	15	—	348
Taco Bravo	1	319	14	42	—	658
Taco Burger	1	281	14	31	—	660
Taco Salad w/ 2 oz Dressing	1	359	24	35	—	790
Taco Salad w/o Dressing	1	228	13	30	—	440
TCBY						
Nonfat, All Flavors	1 giant (31.6 fl oz)	869	tr	182	<5	356
Nonfat, All Flavors	1 super (15.2 fl oz)	418	tr	87	<5	171
Nonfat, All Flavors	1 lg (10.5 fl oz)	289	tr	60	<5	118

FOOD	PORTION	CAL	FAT	CARB	CHOL	SOD
Nonfat, All Flavors	1 reg (8.2 fl oz)	226	tr	47	<5	92
Nonfat, All Flavors	1 sm (5.9 fl oz)	162	tr	34	<5	66
Nonfat, All Flavors	1 kiddie (3.2 fl oz)	88	tr	18	<5	36
Regular, All Flavors	1 giant (31.6 fl oz)	1027	24	182	79	474
Regular, All Flavors	1 super (15.2 fl oz)	494	11	87	38	228
Regular, All Flavors	1 lg (10.5 fl oz)	341	8	60	26	158
Regular, All Flavors	1 sm (5.9 fl oz)	192	4	34	15	89
Regular, All Flavors	1 kiddie (3.2 fl oz)	104	2	18	8	48
Sugar Free, All Flavors	1 giant (31.6 fl oz)	632	tr	142	<5	316
Sugar Free, All Flavors	1 super (15.2 fl oz)	304	tr	68	<5	152
Sugar Free, All Flavors	1 lg (10.5 fl oz)	210	tr	47	<5	105
Sugar Free, All Flavors	1 reg (8.2 fl oz)	164	tr	37	<5	82
Sugar Free, All Flavors	1 sm (5.9 fl oz)	118	tr	26	<5	59
Sugar Free, All Flavors	1 kiddie (3.2 fl oz)	64	tr	14	<5	32

TGI FRIDAY'S

FOOD	PORTION	CAL	FAT	CARB	CHOL	SOD
Charbroiled Chicken Sandwich	1 (7.58 oz)	320	4	37	35	355
Garden Burger	1 (7.58 oz)	410	8	62	10	645
Herb Grilled Chicken	1 (17.72 oz)	550	12	50	110	905
Manicotti	1 serv (15.44 oz)	680	35	53	160	1230

FOOD	PORTION	CAL	FAT	CARB	CHOL	SOD
P&E Shrimp	1 serv (4.38 oz)	120	tr	9	200	670
P.C. Tuna	1 (16.33 oz)	280	7	28	25	740
Pea Salsa	1 (6.35 oz)	170	2	32	0	445
Spinach Salad	1 (8.67 oz)	240	11	21	205	390
Turkey Burger	1 (9.81 oz)	410	19	27	95	780
Vegetable Bagette	1 (16.1 oz)	440	11	71	tr	550
Vegetable Medley	1 serv (13.8 oz)	140	3	17	5	160

T.J. CINNAMON'S

FOOD	PORTION	CAL	FAT	CARB	CHOL	SOD
Doughnuts, Cake	2	454	22	60	98	582
Doughnuts, Raised	2	352	22	32	98	198
Mini-Cinn, Plain	1	75	5	7	3	89
Mini-Cinn w/ Icing	1	80	5	8	3	89
Original Gourmet Cinnamon Roll, Plain	1	630	34	75	38	712
Original Gourmet Cinnamon Roll w/ Icing	1	686	34	89	38	712
Petite Cinnamon Roll, Plain	1	185	10	22	11	214
Petite Cinnamon Roll w/ Icing	1	202	10	26	11	214
Sticky Bun, Cinnamon Pecan	1	607	35	69	29	589
Sticky Bun Petite, Cinnamon Pecan	1	255	15	29	11	241
Triple Chocolate Classic Roll, Plain	1	412	28	35	28	543
Triple Chocolate Classic Roll w/ Icing	1	462	31	42	28	563

FOOD	PORTION	CAL	FAT	CARB	CHOL	SOD

UNO RESTAURANT

| Deep-Dish Pizza | 1 serv | 770 | 38 | 75 | 45 | 1390 |

VILLAGE INN

Cinnamon Raisin French Toast	1 serv	809	16	—	9	740
Fruit & Nut Pancakes, Low Cholesterol	1 serv	936	19	—	2	754
Omelette, Chicken & Cheese	1 serv	721	19	—	120	705
Omelette, Fresh Veggie	1 serv	704	18	—	102	883
Omelette, Mushroom & Cheese	1 serv	680	18	—	102	688
Turkey & Vegetable Scrambled Sensation	1 serv	726	19	—	124	710

WENDY'S

BEVERAGES

Coffee, Decaffeinated Black	1 cup (6 fl oz)	0	0	1	0	0
Coffee, Black	1 cup (6 fl oz)	0	0	1	0	0
Cola	1 sm (8 fl oz)	90	0	24	0	10
Diet Cola	1 sm (8 fl oz)	0	0	0	0	20
Hot Chocolate	1 cup (6 fl oz)	92	1	19	0	120
Lemonade	1 sm (8 fl oz)	90	0	24	0	5
Lemon-Lime	1 sm (8 fl oz)	90	0	24	0	25
Milk, 2%	1 (8 fl oz)	110	4	11	15	115
Tea, Hot	1 cup (6 fl oz)	0	0	0	0	0
Tea, Iced	1 cup (6 fl oz)	0	0	0	0	0

CHILDREN'S MENU SELECTIONS

| Kid's Meal Cheeseburger | 1 (4.3 oz) | 310 | 13 | 33 | 45 | 770 |

FOOD	PORTION	CAL	FAT	CARB	CHOL	SOD
Kid's Meal Hamburger	1 (3.9 oz)	270	9	33	35	600
DESSERTS						
Chocolate Chip Cookie	1 (2.2 oz)	280	13	39	15	260
Frosty Dairy Dessert	1 lg (20 fl oz)	570	17	79	70	330
Frosty Dairy Dessert	1 med (16 fl oz)	460	13	63	55	260
Frosty Dairy Dessert	1 sm (12 fl oz)	340	10	57	40	200
MAIN MENU SELECTIONS						
American Cheese	1 slice (0.6 oz)	70	6	0	15	260
American Cheese Jr.	1 slice (0.4 oz)	45	4	0	10	170
Bacon	1 strip (0.2 oz)	30	3	0	5	125
Baked Potato	1 lg (12 oz)	290	9	31	60	1000
Baked Potato	1 sm (8 oz)	190	6	20	40	670
Baked Potato w/ Bacon & Cheese	1 (13.3 oz)	530	18	77	20	1280
Baked Potato w/ Broccoli & Cheese	1 (14.4 oz)	460	14	79	0	440
Baked Potato w/ Cheese	1 (13.4 oz)	560	23	77	30	610
Baked Potato w/ Chili & Cheese	1 (4.8 oz)	610	24	82	45	700
Baked Potato, Plain	1 (10 oz)	310	0	71	0	25
Baked Potato w/ Sour Cream & Chives	1 (11 oz)	380	6	74	15	40
Big Bacon Classic	1 (10.1 oz)	640	36	44	110	1500
Breaded Chicken Fillet w/o Bun	1 (3.5 oz)	220	10	11	55	400
Breaded Chicken Sandwich	1 (7.3 oz)	450	20	44	60	740
Cheddar Cheese, Shredded	2 tbsp (0.6 oz)	70	6	1	15	110
Chicken Club Sandwich	1 (7.7 oz)	520	25	44	75	990

FOOD	PORTION	CAL	FAT	CARB	CHOL	SOD
Chicken Nuggets	6 pieces (3.3 oz)	280	20	12	50	600
French Fries	1 Biggie (6 oz)	450	22	62	0	280
French Fries	1 med serv (4.8 oz)	360	17	50	0	220
French Fries	1 sm serv (3.2 oz)	240	12	33	0	150
Grilled Chicken Breast w/o Bun	1 (2.5 oz)	100	3	0	50	380
Grilled Chicken Sandwich	1 (6.2 oz)	290	7	35	55	720
Honey Mustard, Reduced Calorie	1 tsp (0.2 oz)	25	2	2	0	45
Jr. Bacon Cheeseburger	1 (6 oz)	440	25	33	65	870
Jr. Cheeseburger	1 (4.5 oz)	320	13	34	45	770
Jr. Cheeseburger Deluxe	1 (6.3 oz)	390	20	36	50	820
Jr. Hamburger	1 (4.1 oz)	270	9	34	35	600
Jr. Hamburger Patty w/o Bun	1 (1.3 oz)	90	6	0	35	110
Kaiser Bun	1 (2.4 oz)	190	3	36	0	340
Ketchup	1 tsp (0.2 oz)	10	0	2	0	95
Lettuce	1 leaf (0.5 oz)	0	0	0	0	0
Mayonnaise	1½ tsp (0.3 oz)	70	7	0	5	45
Mustard	½ tsp (0.2 oz)	5	0	0	0	65
Nuggets Sauce						
Barbeque	1 pkg (1 oz)	50	0	11	0	100
Honey	1 pkg (0.5 oz)	45	0	12	0	0
Sweet & Sour	1 pkg (1 oz)	45	0	11	0	55
Sweet Mustard	1 pkg (1 oz)	50	1	9	0	140
Onion	4 rings (0.5 oz)	0	0	1	0	0
Pickles	4 slices (0.4 oz)	0	0	0	0	140

FOOD	PORTION	CAL	FAT	CARB	CHOL	SOD
Quarter-Pound Hamburger Patty w/o Bun	1 (2.3 oz)	190	12	0	70	220
Saltines	2 (0.2 oz)	25	1	4	0	80
Sandwich Bun	1 (2 oz)	160	3	29	0	280
Single, Plain	1 (4.7 oz)	350	15	31	70	510
Single w/ Everything	1 (7.7 oz)	440	23	36	75	860
Sour Cream	1 pkg (1 oz)	60	6	1	10	15
Tomatoes	1 slice (0.9 oz)	5	0	1	0	0
Whipped Margarine	1 pkg (0.5 oz)	60	5	0	0	105
SALAD DRESSINGS Blue Cheese	2 tbsp (1 oz)	180	19	1	15	180
Blue Cheese, Reduced Calorie, Reduced Fat	2 tbsp (1 oz)	70	7	2	15	260
Celery Seed	2 tbsp (1 oz)	60	7	10	10	220
French	2 tbsp (1 oz)	120	11	7	0	300
French, Fat Free	2 tbsp (1 oz)	35	0	8	0	180
French, Sweet Red	2 tbsp (1 oz)	130	10	10	0	250
Hidden Valley Ranch	2 tbsp (1 oz)	90	10	1	10	210
Italian, Caesar	2 tbsp (1 oz)	150	16	0	15	230
Italian, Golden	2 tbsp (1 oz)	90	7	6	0	450
Italian, Reduced Calorie, Reduced Fat	2 tbsp (1 oz)	40	3	3	0	330
Salad Oil	1 tbsp (0.5 oz)	130	14	0	0	0
Thousand Island	2 tbsp (1 oz)	130	13	4	10	160
Wine Vinegar	1 tbsp (0.5 oz)	0	0	0	0	0
SALADS AND SALAD BAR Alfredo Sauce	¼ cup (1.4 oz)	30	2	4	0	250
Applesauce, Chunky	2 tbsp (1.4 oz)	30	0	7	0	0
Bacon Bits	2 tbsp (0.5 oz)	40	2	1	5	540
Breadstick, Sesame	1	15	0	2	0	20

FOOD	PORTION	CAL	FAT	CARB	CHOL	SOD
Broccoli	¼ cup (0.5 oz)	0	0	1	0	0
Caesar Side Salad	1 (3.1 oz)	110	5	7	15	580
Cantaloupe	1 piece (1.6 oz)	15	0	4	0	0
Carrots	¼ cup (0.6 oz)	5	0	2	0	5
Cauliflower	¼ cup	0	0	1	0	0
Cheddar Chips	2 tbsp (0.4 oz)	70	4	5	0	200
Cheese Sauce	¼ cup (1.2 oz)	25	1	3	0	190
Cheese, Shredded Imitation	2 tbsp (0.6 oz)	50	4	1	0	230
Chicken Salad	2 tbsp (1.2 oz)	70	5	2	0	135
Chives	1 tbsp (1 g)	0	0	1	0	0
Chow Mein Noodles	¼ cup (0.2 oz)	35	2	4	0	30
Coleslaw	2 tbsp (1.3 oz)	45	3	5	5	650
Cottage Cheese	2 tbsp (1.1 oz)	30	2	1	5	125
Croutons	2 tbsp (0.2 oz)	30	1	4	0	75
Cucumbers	2 slices (0.5 oz)	0	0	0	0	0
Eggs, Hard Cooked	2 tbsp (0.9 oz)	40	3	0	110	30
Garden Salad, Deluxe	1 (9.5 oz)	110	6	10	0	320
Green Peas	2 tbsp (0.7 oz)	15	0	3	0	25
Green Peppers	2 pieces (0.3 oz)	8	0	1	0	0
Grilled Chicken Salad	1 (11.9 oz)	200	8	10	50	690
Honeydew Melon	1 piece (1.8 oz)	20	0	5	0	5
Jalapeno Peppers	1 tbsp (0.4 oz)	0	0	1	0	160
Lettuce, Iceberg/ Romaine	1 cup (2.6 oz)	10	0	2	0	5
Macaroni & Cheese	½ cup (3.2 oz)	130	6	14	5	320
Mushrooms	¼ cup (0.5 oz)	0	0	1	0	0
Olives, Black	2 tbsp (0.5 oz)	15	2	1	0	120
Orange Sections	1 (1.1 oz)	10	0	5	0	0
Parmesan Cheese	2 tbsp (0.5 oz)	70	5	1	15	220
Pasta Salad	2 tbsp (1.2 oz)	35	0	3	0	75

FOOD	PORTION	CAL	FAT	CARB	CHOL	SOD
Peaches, Sliced	1 piece (1 oz)	15	0	4	0	0
Pepperoni, Sliced	6 slices (0.2 oz)	30	3	0	5	70
Picante Sauce	2 tbsp (1 oz)	10	0	2	0	260
Pineapple Chunks	4 (1.1 oz)	20	0	5	0	0
Potato Salad	2 tbsp (1.3 oz)	80	7	5	5	180
Pudding, Chocolate	¼ cup (1.8 oz)	70	3	10	0	60
Pudding, Vanilla	¼ cup (1.8 oz)	70	3	10	0	60
Red Onions	3 rings (0.5 oz)	0	0	1	0	0
Red Peppers, Crushed	1 tbsp (0.2 oz)	15	1	3	0	0
Refried Beans	¼ cup (1.9 oz)	80	3	14	0	300
Rotini	½ cup (1.9 oz)	90	2	15	0	—
Seafood Salad	¼ cup (1.3 oz)	70	4	5	0	300
Side Salad	1 (5.4 oz)	60	3	5	0	160
Soft Breadstick	1 (1.5 oz)	130	3	24	5	250
Sour Topping	2 tbsp (1 oz)	60	5	2	0	30
Spaghetti Meat Sauce	¼ cup (1.4 oz)	45	2	6	5	230
Spaghetti Sauce	¼ cup (1.5 oz)	30	0	6	0	340
Spanish Rice	¼ cup (1.8 oz)	60	1	11	0	390
Strawberries	1 (0.9 oz)	10	0	2	0	0
Strawberry Banana Dessert	¼ cup (1.6 oz)	30	0	8	0	0
Sunflower Seeds & Raisins	2 tbsp (0.5 oz)	80	5	5	0	0
Taco Chips	8 (0.9 oz)	120	7	14	0	90
Taco Meat	2 tbsp (1.3 oz)	80	4	2	15	200
Taco Salad	1 (17.9 oz)	580	30	51	75	1060
Taco Sauce	2 tbsp (0.8 oz)	10	0	2	0	110
Taco Shell	1 (0.4 oz)	60	4	6	0	15
Tomato Wedge	1 piece (0.9 oz)	5	0	1	0	0
Tortilla, Flour	1 (1.2 oz)	110	3	18	0	210

FOOD	PORTION	CAL	FAT	CARB	CHOL	SOD
Turkey Ham, Diced	2 tbsp (0.8 oz)	50	4	0	25	280
Watermelon	1 piece (2.2 oz)	20	0	4	0	0

WHATABURGER

BAKED SELECTIONS

FOOD	PORTION	CAL	FAT	CARB	CHOL	SOD
Apple Turnover	1	215	11	27	0	241
Blueberry Muffin	1	239	8	36	0	538
Buttermilk Biscuit	1	280	13	37	3	509
Cookies						
Chocolate Chunk	1	247	16	28	28	75
Macadamia Nut	1	269	16	31	34	80
Oatmeal Raisin	1	222	4	37	28	70
Peanut Butter	1	262	14	30	39	35
Pecan Danish	1	270	16	28	11	418

BEVERAGES

FOOD	PORTION	CAL	FAT	CARB	CHOL	SOD
Cherry Coke	16 fl oz	151	0	40	0	7
Coca-Cola Classic	16 fl oz	141	0	38	0	13
Coffee	1 sm	5	0	1	0	5
Creamer	1 pkg	10	1	1	0	4
Diet Coke	16 fl oz	1	0	tr	0	17
Dr Pepper	16 fl oz	138	tr	35	0	34
Iced Tea	16 fl oz	3	0	1	0	10
Lemon Juice	1 pkg	1	0	tr	0	1
Milk, 2%	1 serv	113	4	11	18	113
Orange Juice	1 serv	77	tr	18	0	2
Root Beer	16 fl oz	158	0	42	0	17
Shake, Chocolate	1 (12 fl oz)	364	9	61	36	172
Shake, Strawberry	1 (12 fl oz)	352	9	60	35	168
Shake, Vanilla	1 (12 fl oz)	325	10	51	37	172
Sprite	16 fl oz	141	0	32	0	30
Sugar	1 pkg	15	0	4	0	0

FOOD	PORTION	CAL	FAT	CARB	CHOL	SOD
Sweet 'n Low	1 pkg	4	0	1	0	0
BREAKFAST SELECTIONS						
Biscuit w/ Bacon	1	359	20	37	15	730
Biscuit w/ Egg & Cheese	1	434	26	38	202	797
Biscuit w/ Egg, Cheese & Bacon	1	511	33	38	213	1010
Biscuit w/ Egg, Cheese & Sausage	1	601	42	38	236	1081
Biscuit w/ Gravy	1	479	27	48	20	1253
Biscuit w/ Sausage	1	446	29	37	37	794
Breakfast Platter w/ Bacon	1 serv	695	44	54	389	1162
Breakfast Platter w/ Sausage	1 serv	785	53	54	412	1234
Breakfast on a Bun	1	455	28	30	232	886
Breakfast on a Bun, Bacon	1	365	19	29	210	815
Butter	1 pkg	36	4	0	11	42
Egg Omelette Sandwich	1	288	13	29	198	602
Grape Jelly	1 pkg	38	0	9	0	0
Hash Browns	1 serv	150	9	16	0	228
Honey	1 pkg	27	0	7	0	0
Margarine	1 pkg	25	3	0	0	40
Pancake Syrup	1 pkg	169	0	42	0	0
Pancakes	3	259	6	40	0	842
Pancakes w/ Sausage	1 serv	426	21	40	34	1127
Scrambled Eggs	2 eggs	189	15	2	374	211
Strawberry Jam	1 pkg	37	0	9	0	0
MAIN MENU SELECTIONS						
Bacon	1 slice	38	3	0	6	106
Baked Potato	1	310	tr	72	0	23

FOOD	PORTION	CAL	FAT	CARB	CHOL	SOD
Baked Potato w/ Broccoli & Cheese Topping	1	453	10	79	17	636
Baked Potato w/ Cheese Topping	1	510	16	80	22	863
Baked Potato w/ Mushroom Topping	1	360	2	80	0	778
Cheese	1 lg serv	89	7	tr	22	338
Cheese	1 sm serv	46	4	tr	12	176
Club Crackers	1 pkg	31	1	4	0	72
Croutons	1 serv	29	1	5	0	88
Fajita Taco, Beef	1	326	12	34	28	670
Fajita Taco, Chicken	1	272	7	35	33	691
French Fries	1 jr serv	221	12	1	0	146
French Fries	1 lg serv	442	24	49	0	292
French Fries	1 reg serv	332	18	37	0	219
Garden Salad w/o dressing	1	56	1	11	0	32
Grilled Chicken Salad	1 serv	150	1	14	49	434
Grilled Chicken Sandwich	1	442	14	48	66	1103
Grilled Chicken Sandwich w/o Dressing	1	385	9	46	66	989
Grilled Turkey Sandwich	1	439	15	49	46	968
Jalapeno Pepper	1	3	tr	1	0	190
Justaburger	1	276	11	30	34	578
Onion Rings	1 lg serv	493	29	51	0	893
Onion Rings	1 reg serv	329	19	34	0	596
Picante Sauce	1 pkg	5	0	1	0	130
Sour Cream	1 serv (2 oz)	121	12	2	25	30
Steak Sandwich	1	387	12	32	61	1164

FOOD	PORTION	CAL	FAT	CARB	CHOL	SOD
Taquito, Bacon	1 serv	335	16	32	286	761
Taquito, Potato	1 serv	446	22	48	281	883
Taquito, Sausage	1 serv	443	26	32	315	790
Whataburger	1	598	26	61	84	1096
Whataburger, Double Meat	1	823	42	62	168	1298
Whataburger Jr.	1	300	12	35	34	583
Whatacatch	1	475	25	43	32	663
Whatachick'n Deluxe	1	573	27	53	56	1338
Whatachick'n Sandwich	1	501	23	51	40	1122
SALAD DRESSINGS						
French	1 pkg	249	20	16	5	729
Ranch	1 pkg	364	38	4	5	599
Thousand Island	1 pkg	280	27	9	0	399
Vinaigrette Lite	1 pkg	36	2	5	0	878

WHITE CASTLE

FOOD	PORTION	CAL	FAT	CARB	CHOL	SOD
Bun	1	74	tr	—	—	—
Cheese	0.3 oz	31	2	—	—	—
Cheeseburger	1 (2.3 oz)	200	11	16	—	360
Chicken Sandwich	1	186	7	—	—	—
Fish w/o Tartar Sandwich	1	155	5	—	—	—
French Fries	1 reg serv	301	15	—	—	—
Hamburger	1 (2.1 oz)	160	8	15	—	270
Onion Rings	1 reg serv	245	13	—	—	—
Sausage Sandwich	1	196	12	—	—	—
Sausage & Egg Sandwich	1	322	22	—	—	—

FOOD	PORTION	CAL	FAT	CARB	CHOL	SOD
WINCHELL'S DONUTS						
Apple Fritter	1 (4.25 oz)	580	37	59	—	201
Cinnamon Crumb	1 (2 oz)	240	11	34	—	208
Cinnamon Roll	1 (3 oz)	360	21	39	—	179
Glazed Jelly	1 (3 oz)	300	13	43	—	172
Glazed Round	1 (1.75 oz)	210	12	24	—	100
Glazed Twist	1 (1.75 oz)	210	11	26	—	100
Iced Chocolate Bar	1 (2 oz)	220	11	28	—	125
Iced Chocolate Cake	1 (2 oz)	230	10	31	—	218
Iced Chocolate Devil's Food	1 (2 oz)	240	12	31	—	221
Iced Chocolate French	1 (1.89 oz)	220	13	23	—	217
Iced Chocolate Raised	1 (1.75 oz)	210	10	26	—	96
Plain	1 (1.58 oz)	200	11	24	—	211
Plain Donut Hole	1 (0.4 oz)	50	3	5	—	13

PART II

TAKE-OUT FOODS

ALL FAT VALUES ARE GIVEN IN GRAMS (G)
ALL CARBOHYDRATE VALUES ARE GIVEN IN GRAMS
ALL CHOLESTEROL VALUES ARE GIVEN IN MILLIGRAMS (MG)
ALL SODIUM VALUES ARE GIVEN IN MILLIGRAMS
A DASH (—) INDICATES DATA WAS NOT AVAILABLE

FOOD	PORTION	CAL	FAT	CARB	CHOL	SOD
BEANS						
baked	½ cup	190	6	27	6	532
barbecue	3.5 oz	120	tr	26	0	460
four-bean salad	3.5 oz	100	tr	20	0	280
refried	½ cup	43	2	5	2	104
three-bean salad	¾ cup	230	11	31	0	500
BEEF DISHES						
bubble & squeak	5 oz	186	13	16	—	—
cornish pasty	1 (8 oz)	847	52	79	—	—
kabob, indian	1 (5.4 oz)	553	40	2	—	—
kheena	6.7 oz	781	71	1	—	—
koftas	5	280	22	3	—	—
roast beef sandwich, plain	1	346	14	33	52	792
roast beef sandwich w/ cheese	1	402	18	27	77	1634
roast beef submarine sandwich w/ tomato, lettuce & mayonnaise	1	411	13	44	73	845
samosa	2 (4 oz)	652	62	20	—	—
shepherd's pie	6 oz	196	10	15	—	—
steak & kidney pie w/ top crust	1 slice (5 oz)	400	26	23	—	—
steak sandwich w/ tomato, lettuce, salt & mayonnaise	1	459	14	52	73	798
stew	6 oz	208	13	6	—	—
stew w/ vegetables	1 cup	220	11	15	71	292
stroganoff	¾ cup	260	19	43	69	503
swiss steak	4.6 oz	214	9	10	61	139
toad in the hole	1 (4.7 oz)	383	29	23	—	—

FOOD	PORTION	CAL	FAT	CARB	CHOL	SOD

BISCUIT

FOOD	PORTION	CAL	FAT	CARB	CHOL	SOD
buttermilk	1	127	6	17	—	368
plain	1	276	34	13	5	584
w/ egg	1	315	20	24	232	655
w/ egg & bacon	1	457	31	29	353	999
w/ egg & sausage	1	582	39	41	302	1142
w/ egg & steak	1	474	28	37	272	888
w/ egg, cheese & bacon	1	477	31	33	261	1261
w/ ham	1	387	18	44	25	1433
w/ sausage	1	485	32	40	34	1071
w/ steak	1	456	26	44	26	795

BLINTZE

FOOD	PORTION	CAL	FAT	CARB	CHOL	SOD
cheese	2	186	6	18	149	268

BREAD

FOOD	PORTION	CAL	FAT	CARB	CHOL	SOD
chapati, as prep w/ fat	1 (2.5 oz)	230	9	34	—	—
chapati, as prep w/o fat	1 (2.5 oz)	141	1	31	—	—
cornbread	2 in × 2 in (1.4 oz)	107	2	18	28	276
cornstick	1 (1.3 oz)	101	4	13	30	195
nan	1 (6 oz)	571	21	85	—	—
papadams, fried	2 (1.5 oz)	81	4	9	—	—
paratha	1 (4.4 oz)	403	18	54	—	—

CABBAGE

FOOD	PORTION	CAL	FAT	CARB	CHOL	SOD
coleslaw w/ dressing	½ cup	42	2	7	5	14
stuffed cabbage	1 (6 oz)	373	22	18	95	1007
sweet & sour red cabbage	4 oz	61	3	8	—	—

FOOD	PORTION	CAL	FAT	CARB	CHOL	SOD
vinegar & oil coleslaw	3.5 oz	150	9	16	0	480

CAKE

FOOD	PORTION	CAL	FAT	CARB	CHOL	SOD
baklava	1 oz	126	9	10	23	78
strudel	1 piece (4.1 oz)	272	8	50	39	142
trifle w/ cream	6 oz	291	16	34	—	—

CHEESE DISHES

FOOD	PORTION	CAL	FAT	CARB	CHOL	SOD
cheese omelette, as prep w/ 2 eggs	1 (6.8 oz)	519	44	31	—	—
fondue	½ cup	303	18	5	62	194
macaroni & cheese	6.3 oz	320	19	25	—	—

CHICKEN

FOOD	PORTION	CAL	FAT	CARB	CHOL	SOD
boneless, breaded & fried w/ barbecue sauce	6 pieces (4.6 oz)	330	18	25	61	830
boneless, breaded & fried w/ honey	6 pieces (4 oz)	339	18	27	61	537
boneless, breaded & fried w/ mustard sauce	6 pieces (4.6 oz)	323	17	21	62	791
boneless, breaded & fried w/ sweet & sour sauce	6 pieces (4.6 oz)	346	18	29	61	791
breast & wing, breaded & fried	2 pieces (5.7 oz)	494	30	20	149	975
drumstick, breaded & fried	2 pieces (5.2 oz)	430	27	16	165	756
thigh, breaded & fried	2 pieces (5.2 oz)	430	27	16	165	756

CHICKEN DISHES

FOOD	PORTION	CAL	FAT	CARB	CHOL	SOD
chicken & dumplings	¾ cup	256	12	12	109	1283

FOOD	PORTION	CAL	FAT	CARB	CHOL	SOD
chicken cacciatore	¾ cup	394	24	9	99	671
chicken paprikash	1½ cups	296	10	—	90	—
chicken pie w/ top crust	1 slice (5.6 oz)	472	31	32	—	—
fillet sandwich, plain	1	515	29	39	60	957
fillet sandwich w/ cheese, lettuce, mayonnaise & tomato	1	632	39	42	76	1238

CHILI

FOOD	PORTION	CAL	FAT	CARB	CHOL	SOD
con carne w/ beans	8.9 oz	254	8	22	133	1008

CLAMS

FOOD	PORTION	CAL	FAT	CARB	CHOL	SOD
breaded & fried	¾ cup	451	26	39	87	833

COFFEE

FAST FACT
Coffee Bars are a new snacking option for the '90s. You'll find them in malls and tucked in a corner of your local bookstore. An espresso, cappuccino or cafe au lait is a pleasant pick-me-up. The Specialty Coffee Association predicts that by 1999 there will be more than 10,000 coffee bars, up from 200 in 1989.

FOOD	PORTION	CAL	FAT	CARB	CHOL	SOD
cafe au lait	1 cup (8 fl oz)	77	4	6	17	62
cafe brulot	1 cup (4.8 fl oz)	48	0	3	0	2
cafe con leche	1 cup (8 fl oz)	77	4	6	17	62
espresso	1 cup (3 fl oz)	2	0	tr	0	2
irish coffee	1 serv (9 fl oz)	107	3	3	12	25
mocha	1 mug (9.6 fl oz)	202	15	17	40	28

CORN

FOOD	PORTION	CAL	FAT	CARB	CHOL	SOD
fritters	1 (1 oz)	62	2	9	12	126

FOOD	PORTION	CAL	FAT	CARB	CHOL	SOD
scalloped	½ cup	258	7	43	47	246

CRAB

FOOD	PORTION	CAL	FAT	CARB	CHOL	SOD
baked	1 (3.8 oz)	160	2	4	184	550
cake	1 (2 oz)	160	10	5	82	492
soft-shell, fried	1 (4.4 oz)	334	18	31	45	1118

CROISSANT

FOOD	PORTION	CAL	FAT	CARB	CHOL	SOD
w/ egg & cheese	1	369	25	24	216	551
w/ egg, cheese & bacon	1	413	28	24	215	889
w/ egg, cheese & ham	1	475	34	24	213	1080
w/ egg, cheese & sausage	1	524	38	25	216	1115

CUCUMBER

FOOD	PORTION	CAL	FAT	CARB	CHOL	SOD
salad	3.5 oz	50	tr	11	0	480

EGG DISHES

FOOD	PORTION	CAL	FAT	CARB	CHOL	SOD
salad	½ cup	307	28	2	562	565
sandwich w/ cheese	1	340	19	26	291	804
sandwich w/ cheese & ham	1	348	16	31	245	1005
scotch egg	1 (4.2 oz)	301	21	16	—	—

EGGPLANT

FOOD	PORTION	CAL	FAT	CARB	CHOL	SOD
baba ghanouj	¼ cup	55	4	5	0	95

ENGLISH MUFFIN

FOOD	PORTION	CAL	FAT	CARB	CHOL	SOD
w/ butter	1	189	6	30	13	386
w/ cheese & sausage	1	394	24	29	58	1036
w/ egg, cheese & bacon	1	487	31	31	274	1135

FOOD	PORTION	CAL	FAT	CARB	CHOL	SOD
w/ egg, cheese & canadian bacon	1	383	20	31	234	785

FISH

kedgeree	5.6 oz	242	11	15	—	—
sandwich w/ tartar sauce	1	431	55	41	—	615
sandwich w/ tartar sauce & cheese	1	524	29	48	68	939
taramasalata	3.5 oz	446	46	4	—	—

FLATFISH

battered & fried	3.2 oz	211	11	15	31	484
breaded & fried	3.2 oz	211	11	15	31	484

FRENCH TOAST

w/ butter	2 slices	356	19	36	117	513

HAMBURGER

double patty w/ bun	1 reg	544	28	43	99	554
double patty w/ cheese & bun	1 reg	457	28	22	110	635
double patty w/ cheese & double bun	1 reg	461	22	44	80	892
double patty w/ cheese, ketchup, mayonnaise, mustard, pickle, tomato & bun	1 lg	706	44	40	141	1149
double patty w/ cheese, ketchup, mayonnaise, onion, pickle, tomato & bun	1 reg	416	21	35	60	1051
double patty w/ ketchup, mayonnaise, mustard, onion, pickle, tomato & bun	1 lg	540	27	40	122	791

FOOD	PORTION	CAL	FAT	CARB	CHOL	SOD
double patty w/ ketchup, mayonnaise, onion, pickle, tomato & bun	1 reg	649	35	53	94	920
double patty w/ ketchup, mustard, onion, pickle & bun	1 reg	576	32	39	102	742
single patty w/ bacon, cheese, ketchup, mustard, onion, pickle & bun	1 lg	609	37	37	112	1044
single patty w/ bun	1 lg	400	23	25	71	474
single patty w/ bun	1 reg	275	12	31	36	387
single patty w/ cheese & bun	1 lg	608	33	47	96	1589
single patty w/ cheese & bun	1 reg	320	15	32	50	500
single patty w/ cheese, ham, ketchup, mayonnaise, pickle, tomato & bun	1 lg	745	48	38	122	1713
single patty w/ ketchup, mayonnaise, mustard, onion, pickle, tomato & bun	1 reg	279	13	27	26	504
triple patty w/ cheese & bun	1 lg	769	51	27	161	1211
triple patty w/ ketchup, mustard, pickle & bun	1 lg	693	41	29	142	713

HAM DISHES

sandwich w/ cheese	1	353	15	33	58	772

HOT DOG

chili dog w/ bun	1	297	13	31	51	480
corndog	1	460	19	56	79	972

FOOD	PORTION	CAL	FAT	CARB	CHOL	SOD
plain w/ bun	1	242	15	18	44	671

ICE CREAM AND FROZEN DESSERTS

FOOD	PORTION	CAL	FAT	CARB	CHOL	SOD
caramel sundae	1 (5.4 oz)	303	9	49	25	195
hot fudge sundae	1 (5.4 oz)	284	9	48	21	182
strawberry sundae	1 (5.4 oz)	269	8	45	21	92
vanilla soft-serve ice milk cone	1 (4.6 oz)	164	6	24	28	92

LAMB DISHES

FOOD	PORTION	CAL	FAT	CARB	CHOL	SOD
curry	¾ cup	345	17	22	89	258
moussaka	5.6 oz	312	21	16	—	—
stew	¾ cup	124	5	11	29	140

LOBSTER

FOOD	PORTION	CAL	FAT	CARB	CHOL	SOD
newburg	1 cup	485	27	13	455	127

LUNCHEON MEATS/COLD CUTS

FOOD	PORTION	CAL	FAT	CARB	CHOL	SOD
submarine w/ cheese, ham, salami, lettuce, onion, tomato & oil	1	456	19	51	35	1650

NOODLES

FOOD	PORTION	CAL	FAT	CARB	CHOL	SOD
noodle pudding	½ cup	132	7	11	27	222

ONION

FOOD	PORTION	CAL	FAT	CARB	CHOL	SOD
rings, breaded & fried	8–9	275	16	31	14	430

ORIENTAL FOOD

FOOD	PORTION	CAL	FAT	CARB	CHOL	SOD
chicken teriyaki	¾ cup	399	27	7	92	2190
chop suey w/ pork	1 cup	375	29	29	62	1378
chow mein, pork	1 cup	425	24	21	89	1673

FOOD	PORTION	CAL	FAT	CARB	CHOL	SOD
chow mein, shrimp	1 cup	221	10	21	55	1658
fried rice	6.6 oz	249	6	48	—	—
fried rice w/ egg	6.7 oz	395	20	49	—	—
wonton soup	1 cup	205	3	26	89	322
wonton, fried	½ cup (1 oz)	111	8	8	31	147

OYSTERS

FOOD	PORTION	CAL	FAT	CARB	CHOL	SOD
battered & fried	6 (4.9 oz)	368	18	40	109	677
breaded & fried	6 (4.9 oz)	368	18	40	109	677
eastern, breaded & fried	3 oz	167	11	10	69	355
eastern, breaded & fried	6 med	173	11	10	72	367
oysters rockefeller	3	66	2	5	38	80
stew	1 cup	278	18	15	100	928

PANCAKES

FOOD	PORTION	CAL	FAT	CARB	CHOL	SOD
buckwheat	1 (4-in diam)	55	2	6	20	125
potato	1 (4-in diam)	78	6	4	60	238
w/ butter & syrup	3	519	14	91	57	1103

PASTA DINNERS

FOOD	PORTION	CAL	FAT	CARB	CHOL	SOD
lasagna	1 piece (2.5 × 2.5 in)	374	21	25	107	668
macaroni & cheese	1 cup	230	10	26	24	730
manicotti	¾ cup (6.4 oz)	273	12	28	77	414
rigatoni w/ sausage sauce	¾ cup	260	12	28	59	106
spaghetti w/ meatballs & cheese	1 cup	407	19	38	104	696

PASTA SALAD

FOOD	PORTION	CAL	FAT	CARB	CHOL	SOD
elbow macaroni salad	3.5 oz	160	5	26	0	590

FOOD	PORTION	CAL	FAT	CARB	CHOL	SOD
italian-style pasta salad	3.5 oz	140	7	15	0	480
mustard macaroni salad	3.5 oz	190	10	23	0	560
pasta salad w/ vegetables	3.5 oz	140	4	21	0	210

PEAS

FOOD	PORTION	CAL	FAT	CARB	CHOL	SOD
pea & potato curry	1 serv (7 oz)	284	22	19	—	—
pea curry	1 serv (4.4 oz)	438	42	11	—	—

PIEROGI

FOOD	PORTION	CAL	FAT	CARB	CHOL	SOD
pierogi	¾ cup (4.4 oz)	307	19	24	49	369

PIZZA

FOOD	PORTION	CAL	FAT	CARB	CHOL	SOD
cheese	⅛ of 12-in pie	140	3	21	9	336
cheese	12-in pie	1121	26	164	74	2680
cheese, meat & vegetables	⅛ of 12-in pie	184	5	21	21	382
cheese, meat & vegetables	12-in pie	1472	43	170	165	3054
pepperoni	⅛ of 12-in pie	181	7	20	14	267
pepperoni	12-in pie	1445	56	157	115	2133

PLANTAINS

FOOD	PORTION	CAL	FAT	CARB	CHOL	SOD
ripe, fried	2.8 oz	214	7	38	—	—

POTATO

FOOD	PORTION	CAL	FAT	CARB	CHOL	SOD
au gratin w/ cheese	½ cup	178	10	17	18	548
baked, topped w/ cheese sauce	1	475	29	47	19	381
baked, topped w/ cheese sauce & bacon	1	451	26	44	30	973

FOOD	PORTION	CAL	FAT	CARB	CHOL	SOD
baked, topped w/ cheese sauce & broccoli	1	402	14	47	20	484
baked, topped w/ cheese sauce & chili	1	481	22	56	31	701
baked, topped w/ sour cream & chives	1	394	22	50	23	182
curry	1 serv (6 oz)	292	16	36	—	—
french fried in beef tallow	1 lg serv	358	19	44	20	187
french fried in beef tallow	1 reg serv	237	12	29	13	124
french fried in vegetable oil	1 lg serv	355	19	44	0	187
french fried in vegetable oil	1 reg serv	235	12	29	0	124
hash browns	½ cup	151	9	16	9	290
mashed w/ whole milk & margarine	⅓ cup	66	tr	13	2	182
mustard potato salad	3.5 oz	120	6	16	0	393
potato salad	½ cup	179	10	14	86	661
potato salad	⅓ cup	108	6	13	57	312
potato salad w/ vegetables	3.5 oz	120	3	20	0	390
scalloped	½ cup	127	5	18	7	435

PUDDING

FOOD	PORTION	CAL	FAT	CARB	CHOL	SOD
blancmange	1 serv (4.7 oz)	154	5	25	—	—
bread pudding	1 serv (6.7 oz)	564	18	94	—	—
queen of puddings	1 serv (4.4 oz)	266	10	41	—	—
rice pudding	1 serv (3 oz)	110	4	17	—	—
rice pudding w/ raisins	½ cup	246	6	42	136	270
tapioca	½ cup	169	6	21	111	154

FOOD	PORTION	CAL	FAT	CARB	CHOL	SOD
QUICHE						
cheese	1 slice (3 oz)	283	20	16	—	—
lorraine	1 slice (3 oz)	352	25	18	—	—
mushroom	1 slice (3 oz)	256	18	17	—	—
RICE						
pilaf	½ cup	84	3	11	22	362
risotto	6.6 oz	426	18	65	—	—
spanish	¾ cup	363	27	19	35	1339
SALAD						
chef w/o dressing	1½ cups	386	28	9	244	279
tossed w/o dressing	1½ cups	32	tr	7	0	53
tossed w/o dressing	¾ cup	16	0	3	0	27
tossed w/o dressing w/ cheese & egg	1½ cups	102	6	5	98	119
tossed w/o dressing w/ chicken	1½ cups	105	2	4	72	209
tossed w/o dressing w/ pasta & seafood	1½ cups (14.6 oz)	380	21	32	50	1572
tossed w/o dressing w/ shrimp	1½ cups	107	2	7	180	487
waldorf	½ cup	79	6	6	8	49
SALMON						
salmon cake	1 (3 oz)	241	15	6	104	602
SAUSAGE						
pork	1 link (.5 oz)	48	4	tr	11	168
pork	1 patty (1 oz)	100	8	tr	22	349
SAUSAGE DISHES						
sausage roll	1 (2.3 oz)	311	24	22	—	—

FOOD	PORTION	CAL	FAT	CARB	CHOL	SOD
SCALLOP						
breaded & fried	6 (5 oz)	386	19	38	107	919
SCONE						
cheese	1 (1.75 oz)	182	9	22	—	—
fruit	1 (1.75 oz)	158	5	27	—	—
plain	1 (1.75 oz)	181	7	27	—	—
SHRIMP						
breaded & fried	4 lg	73	4	3	53	103
breaded & fried	3 oz	206	10	10	150	292
breaded & fried	6–8 (6 oz)	454	25	40	201	1447
jambalaya	¾ cup	188	5	26	50	83
SOUP						
gazpacho	1 cup	46	tr	5	0	63
oxtail	5 oz	64	3	7	—	—
SPAGHETTI SAUCE						
bolognese	5 oz	195	15	4	—	—
SPANISH FOOD						
burrito w/ apple	1 lg (5.4 oz)	484	20	73	7	443
burrito w/ apple	1 sm (2.6 oz)	231	10	35	3	211
burrito w/ beans	2 (7.6 oz)	448	14	71	5	986
burrito w/ beans & cheese	2 (6.5 oz)	377	12	55	27	1166
burrito w/ beans & chili peppers	2 (7.2 oz)	413	15	58	33	1043
burrito w/ beans & meat	2 (8.1 oz)	508	18	66	48	1335

FOOD	PORTION	CAL	FAT	CARB	CHOL	SOD
burrito w/ beans, cheese & beef	2 (7.1 oz)	331	13	40	125	990
burrito w/ beans, cheese & chili peppers	2 (11.8 oz)	663	23	85	158	2060
burrito w/ beef	2 (7.7 oz)	523	21	59	65	1492
burrito w/ beef & chili peppers	2 (7.1 oz)	426	17	49	54	1116
burrito w/ beef, cheese & chili peppers	2 (10.7 oz)	634	25	64	170	2091
burrito w/ cherries	1 lg (5.4 oz)	484	20	73	7	443
burrito w/ cherries	1 sm (2.6 oz)	231	10	35	3	211
chimichanga w/ beef	1 (6.1 oz)	425	20	43	9	910
chimichanga w/ beef & cheese	1 (6.4 oz)	443	23	39	51	956
chimichanga w/ beef & red chili peppers	1 (6.7 oz)	424	19	46	9	1169
chimichanga w/ beef, cheese & red chili peppers	1 (6.3 oz)	364	18	38	50	895
enchilada w/ cheese	1 (5.7 oz)	320	19	29	44	784
enchilada w/ cheese & beef	1 (6.7 oz)	324	18	30	40	1320
enchilada w/ eggplant	1	142	5	—	7	—
enchirito w/ cheese, beef & beans	1 (6.8 oz)	344	16	34	49	1251
frijoles w/ cheese	1 cup (5.9 oz)	226	8	29	36	882
nachos w/ cheese	6–8 (4 oz)	345	19	36	18	816
nachos w/ cheese & jalapeno peppers	6–8 (7.2 oz)	607	34	60	83	1736
nachos w/ cheese, beans, ground beef & peppers	6–8 (8.9 oz)	568	31	56	21	1800

FOOD	PORTION	CAL	FAT	CARB	CHOL	SOD
nachos w/ cinnamon & sugar	6–8 (3.8 oz)	592	36	63	39	439
taco	1 sm (6 oz)	370	21	27	57	802
taco salad	1½ cups	279	15	24	44	763
taco salad w/ chili con carne	1½ cups	288	13	27	4	886
tostada w/ beans & cheese	1 (5.1 oz)	223	10	27	30	543
tostada w/ beans, beef & cheese	1 (7.9 oz)	334	17	30	75	870
tostada w/ beef & cheese	1 (5.7 oz)	315	16	23	41	896
tostada w/ guacamole	2 (9.2 oz)	360	23	32	39	789

SUSHI

FOOD	PORTION	CAL	FAT	CARB	CHOL	SOD
california roll	1 piece (0.8 oz)	28	1	4	1	37
kim chi	⅓ cup (5.8 oz)	18	tr	4	0	2143
sashimi	1 serv (6 oz)	198	7	4	63	718
sushi rice	1 cup (5.2 oz)	157	tr	36	0	368
tuna roll	1 piece (0.7 oz)	23	tr	3	3	33
vegetable roll	1 piece (1.2 oz)	27	1	5	0	48
vinegared ginger	⅓ cup (1.6 oz)	48	tr	12	0	6
wasabi	2 tsp (0.3 oz)	5	tr	1	0	124
yellowtail roll	1 piece (0.6 oz)	25	1	3	0	32

TOMATO

FOOD	PORTION	CAL	FAT	CARB	CHOL	SOD
stewed	1 cup	80	3	13	0	460

TUNA DISHES

FOOD	PORTION	CAL	FAT	CARB	CHOL	SOD
tuna salad	1 cup	383	19	19	27	824
tuna salad	3 oz	159	8	8	11	342

FOOD	PORTION	CAL	FAT	CARB	CHOL	SOD
tuna salad submarine sandwich w/ lettuce & oil	1	584	28	55	47	1294

VEAL DISHES

parmigiana	4.2 oz	279	18	6	136	545

VEGETABLES, MIXED

caponata	¼ cup	28	1	—	0	—
curry	1 serv (7.7 oz)	398	33	22	—	—
pakoras	1 (2 oz)	108	5	12	—	—
ratatouille	8.8 oz	190	16	10	—	—
samosa	2 (4 oz)	519	46	25	—	—

PART III

SNACKS

ALL FAT VALUES ARE GIVEN IN GRAMS (G)
ALL CARBOHYDRATE VALUES ARE GIVEN IN GRAMS
ALL CHOLESTEROL VALUES ARE GIVEN IN MILLIGRAMS (MG)
ALL SODIUM VALUES ARE GIVEN IN MILLIGRAMS
A DASH (—) INDICATES DATA WAS NOT AVAILABLE

FOOD	PORTION	CAL	FAT	CARB	CHOL	SOD

BEER AND ALE

FOOD	PORTION	CAL	FAT	CARB	CHOL	SOD
Amstel Light	12 oz	95	0	—	0	—
Anheuser Busch Natural Light	12 oz	110	0	—	0	—
Bud Light	12 oz	108	0	—	0	—
Coors	12 oz	132	0	30	0	10
Coors Extra Gold	12 oz	147	0	32	0	10
Coors Light	12 oz	101	0	13	0	10
Hamm's	12 oz	137	0	12	0	—
Killian's	12 oz	212	0	29	0	10
Michelob Light	12 oz	134	0	—	0	—
Miller Lite	12 oz	96	0	—	0	—
Molson Light	12 oz	109	0	—	0	—
Old Milwaukee	12 oz	145	0	13	0	25
Old Milwaukee Light	12 oz	122	0	9	0	18
Olympia	12 oz	143	0	12	0	—
Pabst	12 oz	143	0	12	0	—
Piels Light	12 oz	136	0	—	0	—
Schaefer	12 oz	138	0	13	0	23
Schaefer Light	12 oz	111	0	13	0	16
Schlitz	12 oz	145	0	13	0	23
Schlitz Light	12 oz	99	0	3	0	9
Schmidts Light	12 oz	96	0	—	0	—
Signature	12 oz	150	0	13	0	21
Stroh	12 oz	142	0	13	0	23
Stroh Light	12 oz	115	0	7	0	11
Winterfest	12 oz	167	0	38	0	11
ale, brown	10 oz	77	0	8	—	—
ale, pale	10 oz	88	0	12	—	—
beer, light	12 oz can	100	0	5	0	10

FOOD	PORTION	CAL	FAT	CARB	CHOL	SOD
beer, regular	12 oz can	146	0	13	0	19
lager	10 oz	80	0	4	—	—
stout	10 oz	102	0	6	—	—
NONALCOHOLIC						
Guiness Kaliber	12 oz	43	0	—	0	—
Hamm's	12 oz	55	0	12	0	—
Pabst	12 oz	55	0	12	0	—
Spirit	12 oz	80	0	16	0	—

CAKE

FOOD	PORTION	CAL	FAT	CARB	CHOL	SOD
READY-TO-EAT						
Apple Puffs (Entenmann's)	1 (3 oz)	280	13	39	—	320
Apple Strudel, Old Fashioned (Entenmann's)	1 serv (1.5 oz)	120	5	17	—	110
Cheese Topped Buns (Entenmann's)	1 (2.3 oz)	240	12	29	—	240
Cheesecake La Creame, Amaretto Almond (Formagg)	2 oz	115	6	—	0	—
Cheesecake La Creame, Pineapple (Formagg)	2 oz	115	6	—	0	—
Cheesecake La Creame, Plain (Formagg)	2 oz	115	6	—	0	—
Cheesecake La Creame, Strawberry (Formagg)	2 oz	115	6	—	0	—
Cinnamon Buns (Entenmann's)	1 (2.1 oz)	230	10	31	—	200
Cinnamon Filbert Ring (Entenmann's)	1 serv (1.5 oz)	190	12	19	—	160
Coffee Cake, Cheese (Entenmann's)	1 serv (1.6 oz)	150	7	20	—	140

FOOD	PORTION	CAL	FAT	CARB	CHOL	SOD
Coffee Cake, Cheese Filled Crumb (Entenmann's)	1 serv (1.4 oz)	130	6	18	—	140
Coffee Cake, Crumb (Entenmann's)	1 serv (1.3 oz)	160	7	21	—	160
Danish Ring (Entenmann's)	1 serv (1.5 oz)	180	10	18	—	160
Danish Ring, Pecan (Entenmann's)	1 serv (1.5 oz)	190	12	19	—	130
Danish Ring, Walnut (Entenmann's)	1 serv (1.5 oz)	190	12	19	—	130
Danish Twist, Lemon (Entenmann's)	1 serv (1.2 oz)	140	7	17	—	140
Danish Twist, Raspberry (Entenmann's)	1 serv (1.2 oz)	140	7	18	—	120
Date Nut Loaf (Thomas')	1 oz	90	2	18	<5	170
Devil's Food Cake, Fudge Iced (Entenmann's)	1 serv (1.2 oz)	130	5	19	—	120
French Crumb Cake, All Butter (Entenmann's)	1 serv (1.6 oz)	180	8	26	—	220
Louisiana Crunch Cake (Entenmann's)	1 serv (1.7 oz)	180	8	27	—	180
Pound Loaf, All Butter (Entenmann's)	1 serv (1 oz)	110	5	15	—	150
Pound Loaf, Sour Cream (Entenmann's)	1 serv (1 oz)	120	7	14	—	90
Thick Fudge Golden Cake (Entenmann's)	1 serv (1.2 oz)	130	6	20	—	120
angel food	1 cake (11.9 oz)	876	3	197	0	2548
angel food	½ cake (1 oz)	73	tr	16	0	212
bakewell tart	1 slice (3 oz)	410	27	39	—	—
battenburg cake	1 slice (2 oz)	204	10	28	—	—

FOOD	PORTION	CAL	FAT	CARB	CHOL	SOD
cheesecake	1/6 cake (2.8 oz)	256	18	20	44	165
cheesecake	1 cake (9-in diam)	3350	213	317	2053	2464
cherry fudge w/ chocolate frosting	1/8 cake (2.5 oz)	187	9	27	—	160
chocolate w/ chocolate frosting	1/8 cake (2.2 oz)	235	11	35	—	213
coffeecake, cheese	1/6 cake (2.7 oz)	258	12	38	—	257
coffeecake, crumb-topped cheese	1/6 cake (2.7 oz)	258	12	38	—	257
coffeecake, crumb-topped cinnamon	1/9 cake (2.2 oz)	263	15	29	20	221
coffeecake, fruit	1/8 cake (1.8 oz)	156	5	26	—	192
crumpets, toasted	2 (4 oz)	119	1	26	—	—
eccles cake	1 slice (2 oz)	285	16	36	—	—
éclair	1 (1.4 oz)	149	10	15	—	—
fruitcake	1 piece (1.5 oz)	139	4	27	2	116
madeira cake	1 slice (1 oz)	98	4	15	—	—
pound cake	1/10 cake (1 oz)	117	6	15	66	119
pound cake	1 slice (1 oz)	110	12	15	100	108
pound cake	1 cake (8½ × 3½ × 3 in)	1935	94	257	1100	1857
pound cake, sour cream	1/10 cake (1 oz)	117	5	16	17	120
sponge	1/12 cake (1.3 oz)	110	1	23	39	93
strudel, apple	1 piece (2.5 oz)	195	8	29	—	191
treacle tart	1 slice (2.5 oz)	258	10	42	—	—
vanilla slice	1 slice (2.5 oz)	248	13	30	—	—
white w/ white frosting	1/16 cake	260	9	42	3	176
white w/ white frosting	1 cake (9-in diam)	4170	148	670	46	2827

FOOD	PORTION	CAL	FAT	CARB	CHOL	SOD
yellow w/ chocolate frosting	1 cake (9-in diam)	3895	175	620	609	3080
yellow w/ chocolate frosting	⅙ cake (2.2 oz)	242	11	36	35	216
yellow w/ vanilla frosting	⅙ cake (2.2 oz)	239	9	38	—	220
SNACK All Butter Pound (Sara Lee)	1	200	11	23	—	190
Apple Delights (Little Debbie)	1 pkg (1.25 oz)	160	8	21	—	105
Apple Light & Fruity (Drake's)	1 (1.2 oz)	90	1	20	0	110
Apple Oatmeal (Lance)	1 pkg (51 g)	200	9	35	10	210
Apple Spice (Little Debbie)	1 pkg (2.2 oz)	300	17	34	tr	200
Banana Slices (Little Debbie)	1 pkg (3 oz)	380	17	52	tr	240
Banana Twins (Little Debbie)	1 pkg (2.2 oz)	280	13	38	tr	170
Be My Valentine (Little Debbie)	1 pkg (2.2 oz)	290	15	37	tr	120
Blueberry Light & Fruity (Drake's)	1 (1.2 oz)	90	1	20	0	95
Butter Cream Filled Cupcake (Tastykake)	1 (32 g)	120	4	20	5	120
Carrot Cake, Deluxe (Sara Lee)	1	180	7	26	—	200
Cherry Cordials (Little Debbie)	1 pkg (1.3 oz)	180	9	23	tr	85
Choco-Cakes (Little Debbie)	1 pkg (2.17 oz)	270	13	37	tr	220
Choc-O-Jel (Little Debbie)	1 pkg (1.16 oz)	170	10	19	tr	100

FOOD	PORTION	CAL	FAT	CARB	CHOL	SOD
Chocolate Chip (Little Debbie)	1 pkg (2.4 oz)	310	16	40	tr	180
Chocolate Cream Filled Cupcake (Tastykake)	1 (34 g)	130	5	21	5	130
Chocolate Cupcake (Tastykake)	1 (30 g)	100	3	19	5	120
Chocolate Fudge Cake (Sara Lee)	1	190	10	24	—	125
Chocolate Slices (Little Debbie)	1 pkg (3 oz)	360	17	48	tr	310
Chocolate Twins (Little Debbie)	1 pkg (2.2 oz)	260	13	35	tr	220
Christmas Tree Cakes (Little Debbie)	1 pkg (1.5 oz)	200	9	27	tr	95
Cinnamon Raisin Light & Fruity (Drake's)	1 (1.2 oz)	90	1	19	0	105
Classic Cheesecake (Sara Lee)	1	200	14	16	—	150
Coconut (Little Debbie)	1 pkg (2.17 oz)	310	18	34	tr	130
Coconut Crunch (Little Debbie)	1 pkg (2 oz)	340	24	24	tr	50
Coconut Rounds (Little Debbie)	1 pkg (1.13 oz)	160	10	18	tr	85
Coffee Cake (Drake's)	1 (1.1 oz)	140	6	38	10	90
Coffee Cake (Little Debbie)	1 pkg (2 oz)	220	6	18	tr	210
Coffee Cake, Apple Cinnamon (Sara Lee)	1	290	13	40	—	270
Coffee Cake, Butter Streusel (Sara Lee)	1	230	12	27	—	270
Coffee Cake, Chocolate Crumb (Drake's)	1 (2.5 oz)	245	9	38	18	206

FOOD	PORTION	CAL	FAT	CARB	CHOL	SOD
Coffee Cake, Cinnamon Crumb (Drake's)	½ cake (1.3 oz)	150	6	22	10	110
Coffee Cake, Pecan (Sara Lee)	1	280	16	30	—	270
Coffee Cake, Small (Drake's)	1 (2 oz)	220	9	33	15	160
Creamies, Banana Treat (Tastykake)	1	138	3	—	—	—
Creamies, Chocolate (Tastykake)	1	174	7	—	—	—
Creamies, Vanilla (Tastykake)	1	182	8	—	—	—
Cup Cake Lights (Hostess)	1 (1.3 oz)	120	2	25	0	160
Devil Cremes (Little Debbie)	1 pkg (1.3 oz)	170	7	7	tr	170
Devil Dog (Drake's)	1 (1.5 oz)	160	6	24	0	135
Devil Slices (Little Debbie)	1 pkg (3 oz)	320	9	—	tr	—
Devil Squares (Little Debbie)	1 pkg (2.2 oz)	300	17	33	tr	135
Dunking Sticks (Lance)	1 (39 g)	190	10	22	5	130
Easter Bunny Cakes (Little Debbie)	1 pkg (2.5 oz)	320	14	46	tr	140
Easter Puffs (Little Debbie)	1 pkg (1.25 oz)	150	4	27	tr	60
Fancy Cakes (Little Debbie)	1 pkg (2.4 oz)	310	15	42	tr	135
Figaroos (Little Debbie)	1 pkg (1.5 oz)	160	4	31	tr	105
Fig Cake (Lance)	1 pkg (60 g)	210	3	43	0	90
Fudge Crispy (Little Debbie)	1 pkg (2.08 oz)	330	20	35	tr	55

FOOD	PORTION	CAL	FAT	CARB	CHOL	SOD
Fudge Rounds (Little Debbie)	1 pkg (1.19 oz)	150	5	23	tr	75
Funny Bones (Drake's)	1 (1.25 oz)	150	8	18	0	110
Golden Cremes (Little Debbie)	1 pkg (1.47 oz)	160	5	27	tr	150
Holiday Cakes, Chocolate (Little Debbie)	1 pkg (2.4 oz)	330	19	37	tr	135
Holiday Cakes, Vanilla (Little Debbie)	1 pkg (2.5 oz)	350	21	39	tr	160
Honey Bun (Lance)	1 (85 g)	330	14	48	0	210
Honeybun, Glazed (Tastykake)	1 pkg (92 g)	360	20	42	0	220
Honeybun, Iced (Tastykake)	1 pkg (92 g)	350	15	50	50	250
Jelly Rolls (Little Debbie)	1 pkg (2.17 oz)	240	9	40	tr	140
Junior Chocolate (Tastykake)	1 pkg (94 g)	340	12	57	60	220
Junior Coconut (Tastykake)	1 pkg (94 g)	300	6	60	50	300
Junior Lemon (Tastykake)	1 pkg (94 g)	310	7	75	75	330
Junior Orange (Tastykake)	1 pkg (94 g)	340	9	61	50	240
Kandy Kake, Chocolate (Tastykake)	1 (19 g)	80	3	13	0	35
Kandy Kake, Coconut (Tastykake)	1 (19 g)	80	4	11	0	40
Kandy Kake, Peanut Butter (Tastykake)	1 (19 g)	90	4	11	5	40
Koffee Kake, Cream Filled (Tastykake)	1 (29 g)	110	4	18	15	80
Koffee Kake Junior (Tastykake)	1 pkg (71 g)	260	8	44	40	210

FOOD	PORTION	CAL	FAT	CARB	CHOL	SOD
Kreme Kup (Tastykake)	1 (25 g)	90	3	15	5	115
Krimpet, Butterscotch (Tastykake)	1 (28 g)	100	1	19	19	85
Krimpet, Jelly (Tastykake)	1 (28 g)	90	1	19	20	80
Krimpet, Strawberry (Tastykake)	1 (28 g)	100	2	20	20	85
Lemon Stix (Little Debbie)	1 pkg (1.5 oz)	220	11	28	tr	60
Marshmallow Supremes (Little Debbie)	1 pkg (1.25 oz)	150	5	25	tr	65
Mint Sprints (Little Debbie)	1 pkg (1.5 oz)	240	15	25	tr	45
Nutty Bar (Little Debbie)	1 pkg (2 oz)	320	19	31	tr	80
Oatmeal Cake (Lance)	1 (57 g)	240	11	35	0	250
Pastry Pocket, Apple (Tastykake)	1 (85 g)	320	18	38	10	220
Pastry Pocket, Cheese (Tastykake)	1 (85 g)	330	19	38	10	230
Pastry Pocket, Cherry (Tastykake)	1 (85 g)	330	17	41	10	230
Pecan Twins (Little Debbie)	1 pkg (2 oz)	220	9	34	tr	170
Pecan Twirls (Lance)	1 pkg (57 g)	220	8	34	0	190
Pecan Twirls (Tastykake)	1 (28 g)	110	1	17	—	75
Pop-Tarts						
Apple Cinnamon	1	210	6	37	0	170
Blueberry	1	210	6	37	0	210
Brown Sugar Cinnamon	1	210	8	33	0	200
Cherry	1	210	6	37	0	220

FOOD	PORTION	CAL	FAT	CARB	CHOL	SOD
Pop-Tarts *(cont.)*						
Chocolate Graham	1	210	6	37	0	220
Frosted Brown Sugar Cinnamon	1	210	7	34	0	190
Frosted Cherry	1	210	5	37	0	220
Frosted Chocolate Vanilla Creme	1	200	5	37	0	230
Frosted Chocolate Fudge	1	200	5	37	0	220
Frosted Grape	1	200	5	37	0	200
Frosted Raspberry	1	200	5	37	0	210
Frosted Strawberry	1	200	5	37	0	190
Strawberry	1	210	6	37	0	200
Pound Cake (Drake's)	1	110	5	16	25	70
Pumpkin Delights (Little Debbie)	1 pkg (1.13 oz)	140	6	22	tr	110
Raisin Cake (Lance)	1 (57 g)	230	10	35	0	200
Ring Ding (Drake's)	1 (1.5 oz)	180	10	23	0	115
Ring Ding, Mint (Drake's)	1 (1.5 oz)	190	11	22	0	115
Royale Chocolate Cupcake (Tastykake)	1 (46 g)	170	7	28	5	130
Snack Cake, Chocolate (Little Debbie)	1 pkg (2.5 oz)	340	20	38	tr	140
Snack Cake, Vanilla (Little Debbie)	1 pkg (2.6 oz)	360	21	40	tr	160
Star Crunch (Little Debbie)	1 pkg (1.08 oz)	150	7	20	tr	75
Sunny Doodle (Drake's)	1 (1 oz)	100	3	16	10	100
Swiss Cake Roll (Little Debbie)	1 pkg (2.17 oz)	270	12	39	tr	130

FOOD	PORTION	CAL	FAT	CARB	CHOL	SOD
Tasty Too Chocolate Cream Filled Cupcake (Tastykake)	1 (32 g)	100	1	21	0	115
Tasty Too Vanilla Cream Filled Cupcake (Tastykake)	1 (32 g)	100	1	21	0	120
Tasty Twists (Tastykake)	1 (4 g)	18	1	3	—	—
Toaster Tart, Apple Cinnamon (Pepperidge Farm)	1	170	7	25	0	120
Toaster Tart, Cheese (Pepperidge Farm)	1	190	10	22	14	180
Toaster Tart, Strawberry (Pepperidge Farm)	1	190	7	28	0	120
Toastettes (Nabisco)						
Apple	1	190	5	36	0	170
Blueberry	1	190	5	35	0	200
Cherry	1	190	5	35	0	200
Frosted Apple	1	190	5	35	0	170
Frosted Blueberry	1	190	0	35	1	200
Frosted Brown Sugar Cinnamon	1	190	5	35	0	180
Frosted Cherry	1	190	5	35	0	200
Frosted Fruit Punch	1	190	5	35	0	200
Frosted Fudge	1	200	5	34	0	280
Frosted Strawberry	1	190	5	35	0	200
Strawberry	1	190	5	35	0	200
Toast-R-Cakes, BlueBerry	1	110	3	18	—	158
Toast-R-Cakes, Bran	1	103	3	18	—	163
Toast-R-Cakes, Corn	1	120	4	19	—	142

FOOD	PORTION	CAL	FAT	CARB	CHOL	SOD
Vanilla Cremes (Little Debbie)	1 pkg (1.3 oz)	160	7	22	tr	140
Yankee Doodle (Drake's)	1 (1 oz)	100	4	16	0	110
Yodel (Drake's)	1 (1 oz)	150	9	16	5	65
devil's food cupcake w/ chocolate frosting	1	120	4	20	19	92
devil's food w/ creme filling	1 (1 oz)	105	4	17	15	105
sponge w/ creme filling	1 (1.5 oz)	155	5	27	7	155
toaster pastry, apple	1 (1.75 oz)	204	5	37	—	218
toaster pastry, blueberry	1 (1.75 oz)	204	5	37	—	218
toaster pastry, brown sugar cinnamon	1 (1.75 oz)	206	7	34	—	212
toaster pastry, cherry	1 (1.75 oz)	204	5	37	—	218
toaster pastry, strawberry	1 (1.75 oz)	204	5	37	—	218

CANDY

FOOD	PORTION	CAL	FAT	CARB	CHOL	SOD
After Eight Dark Chocolate Wafer Thin Mints (Rowntree)	1	35	1	6	—	0
Almond Joy	1 (1.76 oz)	250	14	28	0	70
Alpine White Bar w/ Almonds (Nestle)	1.25 oz	200	13	18	—	30
Baby Ruth	2.2 oz	300	13	40	0	130
Bar None	1 (1.5 oz)	240	14	23	10	50
Bit-O-Honey	1.7 oz	200	4	39	—	125
Breath Savers, Sugar Free Cinnamon	1 candy	2	0	1	0	0
Breath Savers, Sugar Free Peppermint	1 candy	2	0	0	0	0

FOOD	PORTION	CAL	FAT	CARB	CHOL	SOD
Breath Savers, Sugar Free Spearmint	1 candy	2	0	1	0	0
Breath Savers, Sugar Free Wintergreen	1 candy	2	0	1	0	0
Butter Mints (Kraft)	1	8	0	2	0	0
Butterfinger	2.1 oz	280	12	41	0	105
Caramel Nip (Pearson's)	1 oz	120	3	23	—	70
Caramello	1 (1.6 oz)	220	11	28	10	60
Caramels (Kraft)	1	30	1	6	0	25
Caramels, Chocolate (Estee)	1	30	1	5	0	15
Caramels, Vanilla (Estee)	1	30	1	5	0	15
Caroby Almond Bar (Natural Touch)	4 sections (28 g)	150	10	12	—	50
Caroby Milk Bar (Natural Touch)	4 sections (28 g)	150	9	13	—	55
Caroby Milk Free Bar (Natural Touch)	4 sections (28 g)	160	11	11	—	25
Caroby Mint Bar (Natural Touch)	4 sections (28 g)	150	9	13	—	55
Charleston Chew! Chocolate (Pearson's)	½ bar	120	3	—	—	—
Charleston Chew! Strawberry (Pearson's)	½ bar	120	3	—	—	—
Charleston Chew! Vanilla (Pearson's)	½ bar	120	3	—	—	—
Chocolate Bar, Almond (Estee)	2 sq	60	4	4	2	10
Chocolate Bar, Coconut (Estee)	2 sq	60	4	4	2	10
Chocolate Bar, Fruit & Nut (Estee)	2 sq	60	4	4	2	10

FOOD	PORTION	CAL	FAT	CARB	CHOL	SOD
Chocolate Bar, Peanut (Estee)	2 sq	60	4	4	2	10
Chocolate Coated Raisins (Estee)	10	30	1	5	tr	10
Chocolate Covered Cherries (Cella's)	1 oz	126	4	—	tr	—
Chocolate Fudgies (Kraft)	1	35	1	6	0	25
Chocolate Parfait (Pearson's)	1 oz	120	3	23	—	70
Chocolaty Peanut Bar (Lance)	1 (57 g)	320	18	29	0	40
Chunky	1.4 oz	210	12	22	—	20
Coffee Nip (Pearson's)	1 oz	120	3	23	—	70
Coffico Mocha Parfait (Pearson's)	1 oz	120	3	23	—	70
Crunch 'N Munch, Candied (Franklin)	1.25 oz	170	7	28	0	200
Crunch 'N Munch, Caramel (Franklin)	1.25 oz	160	5	28	13	130
Crunch 'N Munch, Maple Walnut (Franklin)	1.25 oz	160	6	28	6	180
Crunch 'N Munch, Toffee (Franklin)	1.25 oz	160	5	28	6	210
Crunch Chocolate Bar (Estee)	2 sq	45	3	4	2	20
Dark Chocolate Bar (Estee)	2 sq	60	5	5	2	0
Dove Dark Chocolate	1 bar (1.3 oz)	200	12	22	0	0
Dove Dark Chocolate	¼ bar (1.5 oz)	230	14	26	0	0
Dove Dark Chocolate Miniatures	7 (1.5 oz)	230	14	26	0	0
Dove Milk Chocolate	¼ bar (1.5 oz)	230	13	25	10	30

FOOD	PORTION	CAL	FAT	CARB	CHOL	SOD
Dove Milk Chocolate Miniatures	7 (1.5 oz)	230	13	25	10	30
Dove Milk Chocolate Miniatures	1 bar (1.3 oz)	200	7	27	5	25
Estee-ets (Estee)	5	35	2	4	tr	10
5th Avenue	1 (2.1 oz)	290	13	39	5	140
Fruit & Nut Bar (Cadbury)	1 oz	150	8	—	—	—
Fruit And Nut Mix (Estee)	4	35	2	3	tr	10
Golden Almond	½ bar	260	17	20	5	35
Golden III	½ bar	250	15	26	10	40
Goobers	1.38 oz	220	13	19	—	15
Gum Drops (Estee)	4	25	0	6	0	0
Gummy Bears (Estee)	3	20	0	4	0	0
Hard Candy (Estee)	2	25	0	6	0	0
Hershey Bar	1 (1.55 oz)	240	14	25	10	40
Hershey Bar w/ Almonds	1 (1.45 oz)	230	14	20	15	55
Hershey's Kisses	9 (1.46 oz)	220	13	23	10	35
Junior Mints	12	120	3	—	—	—
Kit Kat Wafer	1 (1.625 oz)	250	13	29	10	60
Krackel	1 (1.55 oz)	230	13	27	10	80
Laffy Taffy (Beich's)						
Apple Chews	1 oz	110	1	26	—	55
Banana Chews	1 oz	110	1	26	—	55
Grape Chews	1 oz	110	1	26	—	60
Passion Punch Chews	1 oz	110	1	26	—	50
Strawberry Chews	1 oz	110	1	26	—	55
Sweet & Sour Cherry Chews	1 oz	110	1	26	—	55

FOOD	PORTION	CAL	FAT	CARB	CHOL	SOD
Laffy-Taffy *(cont.)*						
Watermelon Chews	1 oz	110	1	26	—	55
Licorice Nip (Pearson's)	1 oz	120	3	23	—	70
Lifesaver Lollipops, All Flavors	1	45	0	—	0	—
Lifesaver, Sugar Free	1 candy	8	0	—	0	—
Lifesaver Holes, Sunshine Fruits	1 candy	2	0	1	0	0
Lifesaver Holes, Tangerine	1 candy	2	0	1	0	0
Lifesavers						
Christmas Lollipops	1	40	0	10	0	0
Easter Pops	1	40	0	10	0	0
Fancy Fruits	1 candy	8	0	2	0	0
Fruit Juicers, Citrus Fruits	1 candy	8	0	2	0	0
Fruit Juicers, Easter Egg-Sortments	1 candy	10	0	2	0	0
Fruit Juicers, Fruit Punch	1 candy	8	0	2	0	0
Fruit Juicers, Grape	1 candy	8	0	2	0	0
Fruit Juicers, Lollipops	1	40	0	10	0	0
Fruit Juicers, Mixed Berries	1 candy	8	0	2	0	0
Fruit Juicers, Strawberry	1 candy	8	0	2	0	0
Gummi Savers, Grape	1 candy	12	0	3	0	0
Gummi Savers, Mixed Berry	1 candy	12	0	3	0	0

FOOD	PORTION	CAL	FAT	CARB	CHOL	SOD
Sunshine Fruits	1 candy	8	0	2	0	0
Tropical Fruits	1 candy	8	0	2	0	0
Valentine Pops	1	40	0	10	0	0
Wild Cherry	1 candy	8	0	2	0	0
Lollipops (Estee)	1	25	0	6	0	0
Lollipops, Sugar Free (Louis Sherry)	1	18	0	—	0	—
M&M's Almond	1.5 oz	220	12	21	5	20
M&M's Almond	1 pkg (1.3 oz)	200	11	24	5	20
M&M's Mint	1.5 oz	200	9	34	5	30
M&M's Mint	1 pkg (1.7 oz)	230	10	30	10	35
M&M's Peanut	1.5 oz	220	11	28	5	20
M&M's Peanut	1 pkg (1.7 oz)	250	13	13	5	25
M&M's Peanut	1 fun-size pkg (0.7 oz)	110	5	25	5	10
M&M's Peanut Butter	1.5 oz	220	11	27	5	90
M&M's Peanut Butter	1 fun-size pkg (0.7 oz)	110	6	12	5	45
M&M's Peanut Butter	1 pkg (1.6 oz)	240	13	30	5	100
M&M's Plain	1.5 oz	200	9	30	5	30
M&M's Plain	1 fun-size pkg (0.7 oz)	100	5	15	5	15
M&M's Plain	½ king-size pkg (1.6 oz)	200	9	32	5	30
M&M's Plain	1 pkg (1.7 oz)	230	10	25	6	35
M&M's Semisweet	0.5 oz	70	4	9	0	0
Mars	1 bar (1.8 oz)	240	13	31	5	85
Mars Almond Bar	2 fun size (1.3 oz)	190	10	23	5	65
Milk Chocolate Bar (Estee)	2 sq	60	4	4	2	10
Milky Way	1 bar (2.1 oz)	280	11	43	5	90

FOOD	PORTION	CAL	FAT	CARB	CHOL	SOD
Milky Way	2 fun size (1.4 oz)	180	7	28	5	60
Milky Way Dark	1 bar (1.8 oz)	220	8	36	5	85
Milky Way Dark	1 fun size (0.7 oz)	90	3	14	0	35
Milky Way Miniature	5 (1.5 oz)	190	7	30	5	65
Mounds	1 (1.9 oz)	260	14	31	0	85
Mr. GoodBar	1 (1.75 oz)	290	19	23	15	20
Munch Bar	1 (1.4 oz)	230	15	17	10	150
NECCO Mint	1	12	tr	—	0	—
Nestle Crunch	1.4 oz	210	10	26	—	35
Nestle Milk Chocolate	1.45 oz	220	13	25	—	25
Nestle Milk Chocolate w/ Almonds	1.45 oz	230	14	22	—	25
Oh Henry!	2 oz	280	14	32	—	85
Party Mints (Kraft)	1	8	0	2	0	0
PB Max (M&M's)	2 (1.6 oz)	240	15	16	5	160
PB Max (M&M's)	2 fun-size pkg (1.2 oz)	180	12	22	0	115
Peanut Bar (Lance)	1 pkg (50 g)	260	14	24	0	80
Peanut Brittle (Estee)	0.25 oz	35	1	5	0	30
Peanut Brittle (Kraft)	1 oz	130	5	20	0	135
Peanut Butter Cups (Estee)	1	40	3	3	tr	20
Popscotch (Lance)	1 pkg (35 g)	160	6	24	0	120
Raisinets	1.38 oz	180	6	28	—	10
Reese's Peanut Butter Cups	1 (1.8 oz)	280	17	26	10	180
Reese's Pieces	1.85 oz	260	11	32	5	90
Rolo Carmels in Milk Chocolate	8 (1.93 oz)	270	12	37	15	110
Skittles	1.5 oz	170	2	38	0	5

FOOD	PORTION	CAL	FAT	CARB	CHOL	SOD
Skittles	1 pkg (2.2 oz)	250	3	155	0	10
Skittles, Original	2 fun-size pkg (1.4 oz)	160	2	36	0	5
Skittles, Tart-N-Tangy	1.5 oz	170	2	38	0	5
Skittles, Tart-N-Tangy	1 bag (2.2 oz)	250	3	55	0	10
Skittles, Tart-N-Tangy	2 fun-size bags (1.4 oz)	160	2	36	0	5
Skittles, Tropical	1.5 oz	170	2	55	0	5
Skittles, Tropical	1 bag (2.2 oz)	250	3	55	0	10
Skittles, Tropical	2 fun-size bags (1.4 oz)	160	2	36	0	5
Skittles, Wild Berry	1.5 oz	170	2	38	0	5
Skittles, Wild Berry	1 bag (2.2 oz)	250	3	55	0	10
Skittles, Wild Berry	2 fun-size bags (1.4 oz)	160	2	36	0	5
Skor Toffee Bar	1 (1.4 oz)	220	14	22	25	125
Snickers	2 fun-size bars (1.4 oz)	190	9	24	5	100
Snickers	1 bar (2.1 oz)	280	14	36	10	150
Snickers Miniatures	4 (1.3 oz)	170	8	22	5	90
Snickers Peanut Butter	1 bar (2 oz)	310	20	28	5	150
Sno-Caps Nonpareils	1 oz	140	5	21	—	0
Solitaires w/ Almonds	½ bag	260	17	20	5	25
Special Dark Sweet Chocolate Bar (Hershey)	1 (1.45)	220	12	25	0	5
Starburst California Fruits	1 stick (2.1 oz)	240	5	20	0	35
Starburst California Fruits	8 pieces (1.4 oz)	160	4	33	0	20
Starburst Strawberry Fruits	1 stick (2.1 oz)	240	5	48	0	35

FOOD	PORTION	CAL	FAT	CARB	CHOL	SOD
Starburst Strawberry Fruits	8 pieces (1.4 oz)	160	3	33	0	20
Starburst Tropical Fruits	1 stick (2.1 oz)	240	5	48	0	35
Starburst Tropical Fruits	8 pieces (1.4 oz)	160	3	33	0	20
Sugar Babies Tidbits	1 pkg	180	2	—	—	—
Sugar Daddy	1 pop	150	1	—	—	—
Symphony Almond w/ Butterchips	1 (1.4 oz)	220	14	20	—	40
Symphony Milk Chocolate	1 (1.4 oz)	220	13	22	10	35
3 Musketeers	2 fun-size bars (1.1 oz)	140	5	25	5	60
Turtles Pecan Caramel Candy (Demet's)	1 (0.6 oz)	90	5	10	—	15
Twix Caramel	1 (1 oz)	140	7	19	0	60
Twix Caramel	1 fun size (0.6 oz)	80	4	10	0	30
Twix Cookies-N-Creme	1 (0.8 oz)	130	8	13	0	45
Twix Fudge N Crunchy	1 (0.7 oz)	110	6	12	0	35
Velamints	1 mint	9	0	—	0	—
Velamints Cocoamint	1 mint	8	0	—	0	—
Whatchamacallit	1 (1.8 oz)	260	13	30	10	130
Y&S Bites, Cherry	1 oz	100	1	23	0	85
Y&S Twizzlers, Strawberry	1 oz	100	1	23	0	95
York Peppermint Patty	1 (1.5 oz)	180	4	34	0	20
boiled sweets	.25 lb	327	0	87	—	—
candied cherries	1 (4 g)	12	tr	3	0	—

FOOD	PORTION	CAL	FAT	CARB	CHOL	SOD
candied citron	1 oz	89	tr	23	0	82
candied lemon peel	1 oz	90	tr	23	0	14
candied orange peel	1 oz	90	tr	23	0	14
candied pineapple slice	1 slice (2 oz)	179	tr	45	0	—
candy corn	1 oz	105	0	27	0	57
caramels, chocolate	1 oz	115	3	22	1	64
caramels, plain	1 oz	115	3	22	1	64
chocolate	1 oz	145	9	16	6	23
chocolate crisp	1 oz	140	7	18	6	46
chocolate w/ almonds	1 oz	150	10	15	5	23
chocolate w/ peanuts	1 oz	155	11	13	5	19
dark chocolate	1 oz	150	10	16	0	5
fruit pastilles	1 tube (1.4 oz)	101	0	25	—	—
fudge, chocolate	1 oz	115	3	21	1	54
fudge, vanilla	1 oz	115	3	21	1	54
gumdrops	1 oz	100	tr	25	0	10
hard candy	1 oz	110	0	28	0	7
jellybeans	1 oz	105	tr	26	0	7
marzipan	3.5 oz	497	25	57	—	5
mint fondant	1 oz	105	0	27	0	57
nougat nut cream	3.5 oz	342	31	58	—	—

CHEWING GUM

FOOD	PORTION	CAL	FAT	CARB	CHOL	SOD
Beech-Nut Cinnamon	1 piece	10	0	2	0	0
Beech-Nut Fruit	1 piece	10	0	2	0	0
Beech-Nut Peppermint	1 piece	10	0	2	0	0
Beech-Nut Spearmint	1 piece	10	0	2	0	0
Big Red	1 piece	10	tr	2	0	0

FOOD	PORTION	CAL	FAT	CARB	CHOL	SOD
Bubble Yum Fruit Juice Variety	1 piece	20	0	7	0	0
Bubble Yum Luscious Lime	1 piece	25	0	7	0	0
Care*Free Sugarless, All Flavors	1 piece	8	0	—	0	—
Care*Free Sugarless Bubble Gum, All Flavors	1 piece	10	0	—	0	—
Extra Sugar Free Cinnamon	1 piece	8	tr	tr	0	0
Extra Sugar Free Spearmint & Peppermint	1 piece	8	tr	tr	0	0
Extra Sugar Free Winter Fresh	1 piece	8	tr	tr	0	0
Freedent Spearmint, Peppermint & Cinnamon	1 piece	10	tr	3	0	0
Fruit Stripe	1 piece	8	0	3	0	0
Fruit Stripe Bubble Gum	1 piece	8	0	2	0	0
Fruit Stripe Variety Pack	1 piece	8	0	2	0	0
Hubba Bubba Bubble Gum, Cola	1 piece	23	tr	6	0	0
Hubba Bubba Bubble Gum, Sugarfree Grape	1 piece	13	tr	tr	0	0
Hubba Bubba Bubble Gum, Sugarfree Original	1 piece	14	tr	tr	0	0
Hubba Bubba Original	1 piece	23	tr	6	0	0
Hubba Bubba, Strawberry, Grape & Raspberry	1 piece	23	tr	6	0	0
Juicy Fruit	1 piece	10	tr	2	0	0

FOOD	PORTION	CAL	FAT	CARB	CHOL	SOD
Swell Bubble Gum	1 piece (3 g)	10	0	2	0	0
Wrigley's Doublemint	1 piece	10	tr	2	0	0
Wrigley's Spearmint	1 piece	10	tr	2	0	0

CHIPS

CORN
Arrowhead Blue Corn Curls	1 oz	120	2	22	0	126
Arrowhead Blue Corn Curls, Unsalted	1 oz	120	2	22	0	2
Arrowhead Yellow Corn Chips	0.75 oz	90	1	18	0	96
Arrowhead Yellow Corn Chips w/ Cheese	0.75 oz	90	2	15	0	94
Fritos	34 (1 oz)	150	10	16	0	220
Fritos Chili Cheese	34 (1 oz)	160	10	15	0	300
Fritos Crisp 'N Thin	18 (1 oz)	160	10	16	0	240
Fritos Dip Size	13 (1 oz)	150	10	16	0	240
Fritos Non-Stop Nacho Cheese	34 (1 oz)	150	9	16	tr	220
Fritos Rowdy Rustlers Bar-B-Q	34 (1 oz)	150	9	17	0	300
Fritos Wild 'N Mild	32 (1 oz)	160	9	16	0	240
Health Valley	1 oz	160	11	13	0	90
Health Valley, No Salt Added	1 oz	160	11	13	0	1
Health Valley w/ Cheddar Cheese	1 oz	160	10	15	2	120
Lance	1 pkg (50 g)	270	17	26	0	350
Lance BBQ	1 pkg (50 g)	260	16	26	0	360
Snyder's	1 oz	160	11	14	0	150
Snyder's BBQ	1 oz	160	11	14	0	200
Snyder's Chili N Cheese	1 oz	160	11	14	0	170

FOOD	PORTION	CAL	FAT	CARB	CHOL	SOD
Weight Watchers Corn Snackers	0.5 oz	60	2	10	—	230
Weight Watchers Corn Snackers Nacho Cheese	0.5 oz	60	2	10	—	270
Wise	1 oz	160	10	15	0	180
Wise Corn Crunchies	1 oz	160	10	15	0	180
Wise Crispy Corn	1 oz	160	10	15	0	125
Wise Crispy Corn Nacho Cheese	1 oz	160	10	16	0	190
MULTIGRAIN Sunchips	12 (1 oz)	150	8	18	0	100
Sunchips French Onion	12 (1 oz)	140	7	18	tr	120
POTATO Cottage Fries, No Salt Added	1 oz	160	11	14	0	5
Eagle	1 oz	150	10	—	0	—
Eagle BBQ Thins	1 oz	150	10	15	0	220
Eagle Ranch Ridged	1 oz	160	10	15	0	220
Eagle Ridged	1 oz	150	10	15	0	220
Eagle Sour Cream & Onion	1 oz	150	10	15	0	240
Eagle Thins	1 oz	150	10	15	0	220
Eagle Kettle Fry						
BBQ Crunchy	1 oz	150	8	16	0	140
Cape Cod	1 oz	150	8	16	0	120
Cape Cod, No Salt	1 oz	150	8	16	0	0
Cape Cod Waves	1 oz	150	8	16	0	120
Cape Cod Waves, No Salt	1 oz	150	8	16	0	0
Dill & Sour Cream	1 oz	150	8	16	0	160
Dill & Sour Cream, No Salt	1 oz	150	8	16	0	15

FOOD	PORTION	CAL	FAT	CARB	CHOL	SOD
Extra Crunchy	1 oz	150	8	16	0	180
Idaho Russet	1 oz	150	8	16	0	180
Louisiana BBQ	1 oz	150	8	16	0	140
Health Valley						
Country Ripple	1 oz	160	10	15	0	60
Country Ripple, No Salt Added	1 oz	160	10	15	0	1
Dip Chips	1 oz	160	10	15	0	60
Dip Chips, No Salt Added	1 oz	160	10	15	0	1
Natural	1 oz	160	10	15	0	60
Natural, No Salt Added	1 oz	160	10	15	0	1
Kelly's	1 oz	150	9	14	0	160
Kelly's Crunchy	1 oz	150	9	17	0	140
Kelly's Rippled	1 oz	150	9	14	0	160
Kelly's Sour Cream n' Onion	1 oz	150	9	15	0	170
Kelly's Unsalted	1 oz	150	10	14	0	5
Lance	1 pkg (32 g)	190	15	12	0	220
Lance BBQ	1 pkg (32 g)	190	12	18	0	270
Lance Cajun Style	1 pkg (32 g)	160	11	16	0	250
Lance Hot Fries	1 pkg (28 g)	160	10	14	0	220
Lance Ripple	1 pkg (32 g)	190	15	12	0	220
Lance Sour Cream & Onion	1 pkg (32 g)	190	12	18	0	390
Lay's	17 (1 oz)	150	10	15	0	170
Lay's Bar-B-Q	17 (1 oz)	150	9	15	0	270
Lay's Cheddar Cheese	17 (1 oz)	150	10	14	tr	300
Lay's Crunch Tators	16 (1 oz)	150	8	17	0	120
Lay's Crunch Tators, Amazin' Cajun	16 (1 oz)	150	8	17	0	150

FOOD	PORTION	CAL	FAT	CARB	CHOL	SOD
Lay's Crunch Tators, Hoppin' Jalapeno	16 (1 oz)	140	7	18	0	200
Lay's Crunch Tators, Mighty Mesquite	16 (1 oz)	150	8	17	0	135
Lay's Crunch Tators, Supreme Sour Cream	16 (1 oz)	150	8	16	0	180
Lay's Flamin' Hot	17 (1 oz)	150	9	15	0	190
Lay's Kansas City Style Bar-B-Q	17 (1 oz)	150	9	15	0	270
Lay's Salt & Vinegar	17 (1 oz)	150	10	14	0	390
Lay's Sour Cream & Onion	17 (1 oz)	160	10	15	tr	220
Lay's Tangy Ranch	17 (1 oz)	160	10	15	0	210
Lay's Unsalted	17 (1 oz)	150	10	15	0	10
Mr. Phipps Tater Crisps, Bar-B-Que	11 (0.5 oz)	60	2	10	0	160
Mr. Phipps Tater Crisps, Original	11 (0.5 oz)	60	2	10	0	130
Mr. Phipps Tater Crisps, Sour Cream 'n Onion	11 (0.5 oz)	60	2	10	0	150
New York Deli	1 oz	160	11	14	0	120
Old Dutch Foods	1 oz	150	9	16	—	160
Old Dutch Foods Augratin	1 oz	150	8	15	—	220
Old Dutch Foods BBQ	1 oz	140	8	16	—	360
Old Dutch Foods Dill Flavored	1 oz	150	8	16	—	340
Old Dutch Foods Onion & Garlic	1 oz	150	9	15	—	420
Old Dutch Foods Ripple	1 oz	150	9	16	—	150
Old Dutch Foods Sour Cream & Onion	1 oz	150	10	15	—	220
Pringle's	1 oz	170	13	—	0	—

FOOD	PORTION	CAL	FAT	CARB	CHOL	SOD
Pringle's Butter 'n Herbs	1 oz	170	13	—	—	—
Pringle's Cheez-ums	1 oz	170	13	—	tr	—
Pringle's Idaho Rippled	1 oz	170	12	—	0	—
Pringle's Idaho Rippled French Onion	1 oz	170	12	—	tr	—
Pringle's Idaho Rippled Taco 'n Cheddar	1 oz	170	12	—	1	—
Pringle's Light	1 oz	150	8	—	0	—
Pringle's Light B-B-Q	1 oz	150	8	—	0	—
Pringle's Rippled	1 oz	170	12	—	—	—
Pringle's Sour Cream & Onion	1 oz	170	12	—	tr	—
Ruffles	18 (1 oz)	150	10	15	0	135
Ruffles Cheddar Cheese & Sour Cream	18 (1 oz)	160	10	15	tr	250
Ruffles Light	18 (1 oz)	130	6	19	0	140
Ruffles Mesquite Grille B-B-Q	18 (1 oz)	160	10	15	0	270
Ruffles Monterey Jack Cheese Flavor Cheese Attack	18 (1 oz)	160	10	14	tr	200
Ruffles Ranch	18 (1 oz)	160	10	15	0	220
Ruffles Sour Cream & Onion	18 (1 oz)	160	10	15	tr	220
Ruffles Sour Cream & Onion Light	18 (1 oz)	130	6	18	tr	190
Snyder's	1 oz	150	10	13	0	130
Snyder's Au Gratin	1 oz	150	10	13	0	180
Snyder's BBQ	1 oz	150	10	13	0	370
Snyder's Cajun	1 oz	150	10	13	0	350

FOOD	PORTION	CAL	FAT	CARB	CHOL	SOD
Snyder's Coney Island	1 oz	150	10	13	0	280
Snyder's Grilled Steak & Onion	1 oz	150	10	13	0	360
Snyder's Hot Chili	1 oz	150	10	13	0	270
Snyder's Kosher Dill	1 oz	150	10	13	0	400
Snyder's No Salt	1 oz	150	10	13	0	0
Snyder's Salt & Vinegar	1 oz	150	10	13	0	200
Snyder's Smokey Bacon	1 oz	150	10	13	0	260
Snyder's Sour Cream & Onion	1 oz	150	10	13	0	190
Snyder's Sour Cream & Onion Unsalted	1 oz	150	10	13	0	10
Snyder's Zesty Italian	1 oz	150	10	13	0	200
Suprimos Cheddar & Jack	1 oz	140	6	17	tr	180
Suprimos Cool Onion	1 oz	140	6	17	tr	170
Weight Watchers Great Snackers, Barbecue	0.5 oz	70	3	10	0	100
Weight Watchers Great Snackers, Cheddar Cheese	0.5 oz	70	3	10	0	130
Weight Watchers Great Snackers, Sour Cream & Onion	0.5 oz	70	3	10	0	140
Wise Natural	1 oz	160	11	14	0	190
Wise Ridgies Barbecue	1 oz	150	10	14	0	240
potato	1 pkg (8 oz)	1217	79	120	0	1347
potato	1 oz	152	10	15	0	168
sticks	1 pkg (1 oz)	148	10	15	0	71
sticks	½ cup	94	6	10	0	45

FOOD	PORTION	CAL	FAT	CARB	CHOL	SOD
TORTILLA						
Doritos Lightly Salted	16 (1 oz)	150	7	18	0	135
Doritos Salsa 'N Cheese	16 (1 oz)	150	8	17	0	180
Eagle	1 oz	150	8	18	0	140
Eagle Nacho	1 oz	150	8	17	0	200
Eagle Ranch	1 oz	150	8	17	0	150
Eagle Restaurant Style	1 oz	150	7	18	0	100
Eagle Strips	1 oz	150	8	18	0	140
Guiltless Gourmet Baked	22–26 (1 oz)	110	1	21	0	119
Hain Sesame	1 oz	140	7	19	0	190
Hain Sesame Cheese	1 oz	160	8	20	<5	270
Hain Sesame, No Salt Added	1 oz	140	7	19	0	<5
Hain Taco Style	1 oz	160	11	15	<5	320
La FAMOUS	1 oz	140	7	18	0	180
La FAMOUS, No Salt Added	1 oz	140	7	18	0	5
Lance Jalapeno Cheese	1 pkg (1.13 oz)	160	8	—	0	—
Lance Nacho	1 pkg (1.13 oz)	160	8	19	0	240
Old El Paso Crispy Corn	16 (1 oz)	150	8	17	0	106
Old El Paso NACHIPS	9 (1 oz)	150	7	18	0	80
Santitas	1 oz	140	7	19	0	50
Santitas Cantina Style	1 oz	140	6	19	0	75
Santitas Cantina Style, Fajita Flavored	1 oz	140	7	19	0	95
Santitas Strips	1 oz	140	7	19	0	65
Snyder's	1 oz	140	7	18	0	130
Snyder's Enchilada	1 oz	140	7	18	0	150

FOOD	PORTION	CAL	FAT	CARB	CHOL	SOD
Snyder's Nacho Cheese	1 oz	140	7	18	0	130
Snyder's No Salt	1 oz	140	7	18	0	0
Snyder's Ranch	1 oz	140	7	18	0	150
Tostitos	11 (1 oz)	140	8	18	0	160
Tostitos Bite Size	16 (1 oz)	150	8	18	0	110
Tostitos Restaurant Style, Lime 'N Chili	7 (1 oz)	150	7	18	0	190
Tostitos Restaurant Style, White Corn	7 (1 oz)	150	6	20	0	75
Tostitos Baked	1 oz	110	1	24	0	140
Tostitos Baked, Cool Ranch	1 oz	130	3	21	0	170
Tostitos Baked, Unsalted	1 oz	110	1	24	0	0
Wise BRAVOS	1 oz	150	8	18	0	180

COOKIES

FOOD	PORTION	CAL	FAT	CARB	CHOL	SOD
READY-TO-EAT						
Almond Crecents (Sunshine)	2	70	3	10	<2	55
Almond Toast (Stella D'Oro)	1	60	1	10	tr	—
Aloha (LU)	1	75	5	—	—	—
Amaranth Cookies (Health Valley)	1	70	3	12	0	30
Angel Bars (Stella D'Oro)	1	80	5	7	tr	—
Angelica Goodies (Stella D'Oro)	1	110	4	16	tr	—
Angel Wings (Stella D'Oro)	1	70	5	7	1	—
Anginetti (Stella D'Oro)	1	30	1	5	tr	—

FOOD	PORTION	CAL	FAT	CARB	CHOL	SOD
Animal Cookies, Candied (Grandma's)	5 (1 oz)	140	6	5	0	80
Animal Crackers (Sunshine)	7	70	2	—	0	60
Animal Crackers (FFV)	9	110	3	12	—	—
Animal Crackers, Barnum's (Nabisco)	5 (0.5 oz)	60	2	11	0	70
Animal Frackers (Frookie)	6	60	2	9	0	25
Anisette Sponge (Stella D'Oro)	1	50	1	10	tr	—
Anisette Toast (Stella D'Oro)	1	50	1	9	tr	—
Anisette Toast, Jumbo (Stella D'Oro)	1	110	1	23	tr	—
Apple Cinnamon Oat Bran (Frookie)	1 lg	120	4	18	0	100
Apple Cinnamon Oat Bran (Frookie)	1	45	2	7	0	35
Apple Fruitins (Frookie)	1	60	1	12	0	25
Apple Newtons (Nabisco)	1 (0.75 oz)	70	2	15	0	70
Apple Newtons, Fat Free (Nabisco)	1 (0.75 oz)	70	0	16	0	45
Apple Pastry, Dietetic (Stella D'Oro)	1	90	4	14	—	<10
Apple Raisin Bar (Weight Watchers)	1	100	3	18	—	115
Arrowroot Biscuit (Nabisco)	1 (0.25 oz)	20	1	3	<2	15
Baked Apple Bar (Sunbelt)	1 pkg (1.31 oz)	130	2	28	—	130
Bakers Bonus Oatmeal (Nabisco)	1 (0.5 oz)	80	3	12	0	65

FOOD	PORTION	CAL	FAT	CARB	CHOL	SOD
Barre Chocolat (LU)	1	65	3	—	—	—
Bavarian Fingers (Sunshine)	1	70	3	10	0	55
Beacon Hill Chocolate Chocolate Walnut (Pepperidge Farm)	1	120	7	14	5	65
Biscos Sugar Wafers (Nabisco)	4 (0.5 oz)	70	3	10	0	20
Biscos Waffle Cremes (Nabisco)	1 (0.25 oz)	40	2	6	0	10
Bordeaux (Pepperidge Farm)	2	70	3	11	0	40
Breakfast Treats (Stella D'Oro)	1	100	4	15	tr	—
Brown Edge Wafers (Nabisco)	2½ (0.5 oz)	70	2	10	<2	45
Brownie Chocolate Nut (Pepperidge Farm)	2	110	7	11	<5	45
Brownie Nut, Large (Pepperidge Farm)	1	140	8	15	5	65
Brussels (Pepperidge Farm)	2	110	5	13	0	65
Brussels Mint (Pepperidge Farm)	2	130	7	17	0	40
Bugs Bunny Graham Cookies (Nabisco)	5 (0.5 oz)	60	2	11	0	70
Butter Chessman (Pepperidge Farm)	2	90	4	12	10	60
Butter Flavored Cookies (Sunshine)	2	60	2	9	<2	55
Buttercup (Keebler)	3	70	3	11	0	110
Cameo (Nabisco)	1 (0.5 oz)	70	3	10	0	50
Cappuccino (Pepperidge Farm)	1	50	3	6	<5	20

FOOD	PORTION	CAL	FAT	CARB	CHOL	SOD
Capri (Pepperidge Farm)	1	80	5	10	0	45
Caramel Patties (FFV)	2	150	7	—	—	—
Castelets (Stella D'Oro)	1	70	3	10	tr	—
Castelets, Chocolate (Stella D'Oro)	1	70	3	10	tr	—
Champagne (Pepperidge Farm)	2	110	6	—	—	—
Chantilly (Pepperidge Farm)	1	80	2	14	<5	35
Chesapeake Chocolate Chunk Pecan (Pepperidge Farm)	1	120	7	14	5	60
Cheyenne Peanut Butter Milk Chocolate Chunk (Pepperidge Farm)	1	110	6	13	5	80
Chinese Dessert Cookies (Stella D'Oro)	1	170	9	20	tr	—
Chip-A-Roos (Sunshine)	1	60	3	7	0	45
Chips Ahoy! (Nabisco)						
Bite Size Chocolate Chip	6 (0.5 oz)	70	3	9	0	50
Chewy Chocolate Chip	1 (0.5 oz)	60	3	8	<2	40
Chocolate Chunk Pecan	1 (0.5 oz)	100	6	10	10	65
Chunky Chocolate Chip	1 (0.5 oz)	90	5	11	10	90
Heath Toffee Chunk	1 (0.5 oz)	90	5	10	5	90
Oatmeal Chocolate Chip	1	90	5	10	<5	50
Real Chocolate Chip	1 (0.5 oz)	50	2	7	0	40

FOOD	PORTION	CAL	FAT	CARB	CHOL	SOD
Chips Ahoy! *(cont.)*						
Rockers Chocolate Chip	1 (0.5 oz)	60	3	8	0	40
Sprinkled Real Chocolate Chip	1 (0.5 oz)	60	3	8	0	40
Striped Chocolate Chip	1 (0.5 oz)	90	5	10	0	45
White Fudge Chunk	1 (0.5 oz)	90	5	10	<5	75
Chips Chocolat (LU)	1	85	5	—	—	—
Chocolate (Weight Watchers)	3	80	3	13	—	135
Chocolate Cookiesaurus (Sunshine)	7	120	5	19	0	140
Chocolate Sandwich (Weight Watchers)	2	90	3	15	0	90
Chocolate Chip (Archway)	1	60	3	—	5	—
Chocolate Chip (Drake's)	2 (1 oz)	140	6	18	0	110
Chocolate Chip (Duncan Hines)	2	110	5	—	—	—
Chocolate Chip (Entenmann's)	3 (0.9 oz)	140	7	19	—	85
Chocolate Chip (Frookie)	1	45	2	7	0	35
Chocolate Chip (Frookie)	1 lg	120	4	18	0	100
Chocolate Chip (Grandma's)	2 (2.75 oz)	370	17	50	5	270
Chocolate Chip (Nutra/Balance)	1 (2 oz)	260	14	34	—	81
Chocolate Chip (Pepperidge Farm)	2	100	5	12	5	45
Chocolate Chip (Weight Watchers)	2	90	2	18	—	65

FOOD	PORTION	CAL	FAT	CARB	CHOL	SOD
Chocolate Chip Bar (Tastykake)	1 (43 g)	190	8	28	5	95
Chocolate Chip Fudge (Lance)	1 (28 g)	130	5	20	5	130
Chocolate Chip, Large (Pepperidge Farm)	1	130	6	16	5	60
Chocolate Chip Mint (Frookie)	1	45	2	7	0	35
Chocolate Chip Rich 'N Chewy (Grandma's)	3 (1 oz)	140	6	20	5	80
Chocolate Chip Snaps (Nabisco)	3 (0.5 oz)	70	2	11	0	50
Chocolate Chip Soft (Lance)	1 (28 g)	130	5	19	5	100
Chocolate Chunk Macadamia Nut (Tastykake)	1 pkg (56 g)	310	14	42	40	180
Chocolate Chunk Pecan (Pepperidge Farm)	1	70	4	8	12	25
Chocolate Fudge Sandwich (Keebler)	1	80	4	12	0	70
Chocolate Snaps (Nabisco)	4 (0.5 oz)	70	2	11	<2	75
Chocolate-Chocolate Chip (Drake's)	2 (1 oz)	130	5	19	0	85
Chocolu (LU)	1	55	3	—	—	—
Choc-O-Lunch (Lance)	1 pkg (37 g)	180	7	26	0	150
Choc-O-Mint (Lance)	1 pkg (35 g)	180	10	22	0	90
Coated Graham (Lance)	1 pkg (50 g)	200	10	24	0	60
Coconut (Drake's)	2 (1 oz)	130	5	20	0	95
Coconut Cookies, Dietetic (Stella D'Oro)	1	50	2	6	—	<10

FOOD	PORTION	CAL	FAT	CARB	CHOL	SOD
Coconut Macaroons (Drake's)	1 (1 oz)	135	7	17	0	80
Coconut Macaroons (Stella D'Oro)	1	60	3	6	tr	—
Commodore (Keebler)	1	60	2	10	0	65
Como Delight (Stella D'Oro)	1	150	7	18	1	—
Cookie Caramel Bars (Little Debbie)	1 pkg (1.17 oz)	170	8	22	tr	85
Cookie Mates (Keebler)	2	50	2	8	0	55
Cookies 'N Fudge, Party Grahams (Nabisco)	1 (0.25 oz)	45	2	6	0	35
Cookies 'N Fudge, Striped (Nabisco)	1 (0.5 oz)	60	3	7	0	60
Cookies 'N Fudge, Striped Wafers (Nabisco)	1 (0.5 oz)	70	4	8	0	25
Craquelin (LU)	1	55	3	—	—	—
Creme Filled Chocolate (Little Debbie)	1 pkg (1.8 oz)	250	12	35	tr	260
Creme Filled Wafers, Assorted (Estee)	1	30	2	4	0	5
Creme Filled Wafers, Chocolate (Estee)	1	20	1	3	0	5
Creme Filled Wafers, Vanilla (Estee)	1	20	1	3	0	5
Crokine (LU)	2	19	0	—	0	—
Dakota Milk Chocolate Oatmeal (Pepperidge Farm)	1	110	6	15	5	70
Danish Imported (Nabisco)	2 (0.5 oz)	70	4	9	0	15
Date Pecan (Pepperidge Farm)	2	110	5	15	10	40

FOOD	PORTION	CAL	FAT	CARB	CHOL	SOD
Devil's Food Cakes (Nabisco)	1 (0.75 oz)	70	1	15	0	40
Dinosaur Grrrahams (Mother's)	1	70	2	12	<2	50
Dinosaur Grrrahams, Chocolate Salerno (Mother's)	1 pkg (1.25 oz)	167	5	25	0	139
Dinosaur Grrrahams, Cinnamon Salerno (Mother's)	1 pkg (1.25 oz)	165	3	26	0	144
Dinosaur Grrrahams, Original Salerno (Mother's)	1 pkg (1.25 oz)	156	3	26	0	114
Dixi Vanilla (Sunshine)	2	130	5	19	0	110
Dunkaroos (General Mills)	1 pkg (1 oz)	130	5	19	0	70
Dutch Apple Bars (Stella D'Oro)	1	110	3	19	1	—
Egg Biscuits, Dietetic (Stella D'Oro)	1	40	1	7	—	<10
Egg Biscuits, Sugared (Stella D'Oro)	1	80	1	14	1	—
Egg, Jumbo (Stella D'Oro)	1	50	1	9	tr	—
Euphrates (LU)	2	40	2	—	—	—
Famous Chocolate Wafers (Nabisco)	2½ (0.5 oz)	70	2	11	<2	100
Fancy Fruit Chunks, Apricot Almond (Health Valley)	2	90	4	12	0	45
Fancy Fruit Chunks, Date Pecan (Health Valley)	2	90	4	13	0	45
Fancy Fruit Chunks, Raisin Oat Bran (Health Valley)	2	70	2	13	0	95

FOOD	PORTION	CAL	FAT	CARB	CHOL	SOD
Fancy Fruit Chunks, Tropical Fruit (Health Valley)	2	90	3	15	0	45
Fancy Peanut Chunks (Health Valley)	2	90	3	12	0	55
Fat-Free Apple Spice (Health Valley)	3	75	tr	17	0	40
Fat-Free Apricot Delight (Health Valley)	3	75	tr	16	0	40
Fat-Free Date Delight (Health Valley)	3	75	tr	17	0	40
Fat-Free Hawaiian Fruit (Health Valley)	3	75	tr	16	0	40
Fat-Free Jumbos, Apple Raisin (Health Valley)	1	70	tr	16	0	35
Fat-Free Jumbos, Raisin (Health Valley)	1	70	tr	16	0	35
Fat-Free Jumbos, Raspberry (Health Valley)	1	70	tr	16	0	35
Fat-Free Raisin Oatmeal (Health Valley)	3	75	tr	17	0	40
Fiber Jumbos, Blueberry Nut (Health Valley)	1	100	3	14	0	45
Fiber Jumbos, Chunky Pecan (Health Valley)	1	100	3	14	0	45
Fiber Jumbos, Raisin Nut (Health Valley)	1	100	3	14	0	45
Fig Bar (Lance)	1 pkg (42 g)	150	2	30	0	85
Fig Bar (Mother's)	1 oz	100	2	20	<2	75
Fig Bar (Sunshine)	1	50	1	10	<2	35
Fig Bar, Vanilla (FFV)	1	60	1	—	—	—

FOOD	PORTION	CAL	FAT	CARB	CHOL	SOD
Fig Bar, Whole Wheat (FFV)	1	60	1	—	—	—
Fig Fruitins (Frookie)	1	60	1	12	0	25
Fig Newtons (Nabisco)	1 (0.5 oz)	60	1	11	0	60
Fig Newtons, Fat Free (Nabisco)	1 (0.75 oz)	70	0	15	0	80
Fig Pastry, Dietetic (Stella D'Oro)	1	95	4	—	—	—
Fortune (La Choy)	1	15	tr	4	0	1
French Vanilla Creme (Keebler)	1	80	4	12	0	80
Fruit & Fitness (Health Valley)	5	200	6	34	0	115
Fruit-Filled, Apricot-Raspberry (Pepperidge Farm)	2	100	4	15	10	50
Fruit-Filled, Strawberry (Pepperidge Farm)	2	100	5	15	10	50
Fruit-Filled Bar, Apple (Weight Watchers)	1	80	tr	21	0	35
Fruit-Filled Bar, Raspberry (Weight Watchers)	1	80	tr	22	0	45
Fruit Jumbos, Almond Date (Health Valley)	1	70	3	10	0	30
Fruit Jumbos, Oat Bran (Health Valley)	1	70	2	12	0	35
Fruit Jumbos, Raisin Nut (Health Valley)	1	70	3	10	0	35
Fruit Jumbos, Tropical Fruit (Health Valley)	1	70	3	10	0	35

FOOD	PORTION	CAL	FAT	CARB	CHOL	SOD
Fruit Slices (Stella D'Oro)	1	60	2	9	tr	—
Fudge (Estee)	1	30	1	4	0	0
Fudge Bar (Tastykake)	1 (50 g)	200	7	35	5	160
Fudge Chips, Chocolate (LU)	1	75	4	—	—	—
Fudge Chocolate Chip (Grandma's)	2 (2.75 oz)	350	13	54	5	380
Fudge Dipped Grahams (Sunshine)	2	80	4	11	<2	40
Fudge Family Bears, Chocolate w/ Vanilla Filling (Sunshine)	1	70	3	9	0	60
Fudge Family Bears, Peanut Butter (Sunshine)	1	70	3	9	0	65
Fudge Family Bears, Vanilla w/ Fudge Filling (Sunshine)	1	60	3	9	0	50
Fudge Striped Shortbread (Sunshine)	3	160	8	21	<2	80
FundaMiddles Vanilla Creme in Chocolate Graham Shells (General Mills)	1 pkg (0.8 oz)	110	4	18	—	120
Gaufrettes (LU)	2	85	4	—	—	—
Geneva (Pepperidge Farm)	2	130	6	14	0	50
Ginger Boys, Calcium Enriched (FFV)	6	120	3	—	—	—
Gingerman (Pepperidge Farm)	2	70	3	10	5	50
Gingersnaps (Archway)	1	35	1	—	0	—
Ginger Snaps (Bakery Wagon)	4–5 (1 oz)	140	6	19	0	105

FOOD	PORTION	CAL	FAT	CARB	CHOL	SOD
Ginger Snaps (Sunshine)	3	60	2	19	0	70
Ginger Snaps, Old Fashioned (Nabisco)	2 (0.5 oz)	60	1	11	0	80
Ginger Spice (Frookie)	1	45	2	7	0	35
Golden Bars (Stella D'Oro)	1	110	4	16	tr	—
Golden Fruit (Sunshine)	1	70	1	14	<2	40
Grab Cookie Bits, Chocolate (Grandma's)	8 (1 oz)	140	6	19	0	180
Grab Cookie Bits, Peanut Butter (Grandma's)	8 (1 oz)	140	6	19	0	125
Grab Cookie Bits, Vanilla (Grandma's)	8 (1 oz)	140	6	20	5	75
Graham (Nabisco)	2 (0.5 oz)	60	1	11	0	90
Graham, Amaranth (Health Valley)	7	110	3	25	0	110
Graham, Chocolate (Nabisco)	1 (0.5 oz)	50	3	7	0	30
Graham, Honey (Health Valley)	7	100	4	18	0	125
Graham, Honey, Fiber Enriched (Keebler)	2	90	2	16	0	110
Graham, Kitchen Rich (Keebler)	2	60	2	9	0	55
Graham, Oat Bran (Health Valley)	7	120	3	20	0	45
Grahamy Bears (Sunshine)	4	60	2	9	0	55
Hazelnut (Pepperidge Farm)	2	110	6	15	0	75
Hermit (Drake's)	1 (2 oz)	230	7	38	10	280

FOOD	PORTION	CAL	FAT	CARB	CHOL	SOD
Heyday, Caramel & Peanut (Nabisco)	1 (0.75 oz)	110	6	13	0	40
Heyday, Fudge (Nabisco)	1 (0.75 oz)	110	6	13	0	40
Holiday Trinkets (Stella D'Oro)	1	40	2	5	tr	—
Homeplate (Keebler)	1	60	2	10	1	130
Honey Jumbos, Crisp Cinnamon (Health Valley)	1	70	4	9	0	35
Honey Jumbos, Crisp Peanut Butter (Health Valley)	1	70	2	11	0	35
Honey Jumbos, Fancy Oat Bran (Health Valley)	2	130	4	20	0	50
Honey Maid Cinnamon (Nabisco)	2 (0.5 oz)	60	1	12	0	85
Honey Maid Grahams (Nabisco)	2 (0.5 oz)	60	1	11	0	90
Hostess Assortment (Stella D'Oro)	1	40	2	6	tr	—
Hydrox	1	50	2	7	0	45
Hydrox Doubles, Peanut Butter	1	60	3	8	0	65
Iced Gingerbread Cookies (Sunshine)	3	70	3	10	<5	75
Ideal Bars, Chocolate & Peanut (Nabisco)	1 (0.75 oz)	90	5	10	0	80
Irish Oatmeal (Pepperidge Farm)	2	90	5	13	5	80
Jelly Tarts (FFV)	2	110	4	—	—	—
Jingles (Sunshine)	3	70	3	11	0	55
Keebies (Keebler)	1	80	3	12	0	80
Kichel, Dietetic (Stella D'Oro)	1	8	1	1	—	<10

FOOD	PORTION	CAL	FAT	CARB	CHOL	SOD
Krisp Kreem Wafers (Keebler)	2	50	3	7	0	20
Lady Stella Assortment (Stella D'Oro)	1	40	2	6	tr	—
Lem-O-Lunch (Lance)	1 pkg (48 g)	240	11	32	0	190
Lemon Coolers (Sunshine)	2	60	2	9	<2	45
Lemon Nekot (Lance)	1 pkg (42 g)	220	11	28	5	100
Lemon Nut Crunch (Pepperidge Farm)	2	110	7	13	<5	50
Le Petit Beurre (LU)	1	40	1	—	—	—
Lido (Pepperidge Farm)	1	90	5	10	<5	30
Linzer (Pepperidge Farm)	1	120	4	20	<5	55
Little Schoolboy (LU)	1	65	3	—	—	—
Lorna Doone (Nabisco)	2 (0.5 oz)	70	4	9	<5	65
Love Cookies (Stella D'Oro)	1	110	5	13	1	—
Mallomars (Nabisco)	1 (0.5 oz)	60	3	9	0	20
Mallopuffs (Sunshine)	1	70	2	12	0	35
Malt (Lance)	1 pkg (35 g)	190	11	16	0	125
Mandarin Chocolate Chip (Frookie)	1	45	2	7	0	35
Margherite, Chocolate (Stella D'Oro)	1	70	3	10	tr	—
Margherite, Vanilla (Stella D'Oro)	1	70	3	10	tr	—
Marie LU (LU)	1	50	2	8	—	45
Marshmallow Puffs (Nabisco)	1 (0.75 oz)	90	4	14	0	40
Marshmallow Twirls (Nabisco)	1 (1 oz)	130	5	20	0	50

FOOD	PORTION	CAL	FAT	CARB	CHOL	SOD
Milano (Pepperidge Farm)	2	120	6	15	15	45
Milk Chocolate Chip (Duncan Hines)	2	110	5	—	—	—
Milk Chocolate Macadamia (Pepperidge Farm)	2	140	8	—	—	—
Milk Lunch (LU)	1	35	1	—	—	—
Mini Chocolate Chip Cookies (Sunshine)	2	70	4	8	0	50
Mint Milano (Pepperidge Farm)	2	150	7	17	5	60
Mint Sandwich (FFV)	2	160	7	—	—	—
Molasses (Archway)	1	100	2	—	10	—
Molasses Crisps (Pepperidge Farm)	2	70	3	8	0	50
Molasses Iced (Bakery Wagon)	1	100	4	17	<2	120
Mystic Mint (Nabisco)	1 (0.5 oz)	90	5	11	<2	65
Nantucket Chocolate Chunk (Pepperidge Farm)	1	120	6	15	5	60
Nassau (Pepperidge Farm)	1	80	5	9	<5	45
Nilla Wafers (Nabisco)	3½ (0.5 oz)	60	2	11	<5	45
Nut-O-Lunch (Lance)	1 oz	140	5	—	0	—
Nutter Butter Bites (Nabisco)	4½ (0.5 oz)	70	3	9	<2	55
Nutter Butter Peanut Butter (Nabisco)	1 (0.5 oz)	70	3	9	<2	50
Nutter Butter Peanut Creme (Nabisco)	2 (0.5 oz)	80	4	8	0	45
Oat Bran Animal Cookies (Health Valley)	7	110	4	17	0	50

FOOD	PORTION	CAL	FAT	CARB	CHOL	SOD
Oat Bran Fruit & Nut (Health Valley)	2	110	4	17	0	70
Oat Bran Muffin (Frookie)	1	45	2	7	0	35
Oat Bran Muffin (Frookie)	1 lg	120	4	18	0	100
Oat Bran w/ Nuts & Raisins (Sunshine)	1	60	3	8	0	55
Oatmeal (Archway)	1	110	3	1	5	—
Oatmeal (Drake's)	2 (1 oz)	120	5	19	0	50
Oatmeal (Lance)	1 (57 g)	130	5	20	0	70
Oatmeal (Little Debbie)	1 pkg (2.75 oz)	340	12	52	tr	440
Oatmeal (Mother's)	1	60	3	8	0	80
Oatmeal, Apple Filled (Archway)	1	90	1	—	5	—
Oatmeal, Apple Spice (Grandma's)	2 (2.75 oz)	330	12	51	10	570
Oatmeal, Calcium Enriched (FFV)	5	130	5	—	—	—
Oatmeal, Country Style (Sunshine)	1	70	3	10	0	65
Oatmeal Creme (Drake's)	1 (2 oz)	240	9	9	2	250
Oatmeal, Date Filled (Archway)	1	100	2	—	5	—
Oatmeal, Date Filled (Bakery Wagon)	1	90	3	15	<2	100
Oatmeal, Large (Pepperidge Farm)	1	120	6	18	5	105
Oatmeal Raisin (Duncan Hines)	2	110	5	—	—	—
Oatmeal Raisin (Nutra/Balance)	1 (2 oz)	240	9	36	—	50

FOOD	PORTION	CAL	FAT	CARB	CHOL	SOD
Oatmeal Raisin (Frookie)	1	45	2	7	0	35
Oatmeal Raisin (Frookie)	1 lg	120	4	18	0	100
Oatmeal Raisin (Pepperidge Farm)	2	110	5	18	10	11
Oatmeal Raisin (Weight Watchers)	2	90	tr	20	0	75
Oatmeal Raisin Bar (Tastykake)	1 (50 g)	210	8	32	15	250
Oatmeal, Soft (Bakery Wagon)	1	100	5	15	<2	105
Oatmeal Spice (Weight Watchers)	3	80	2	13	—	75
Old-Fashion Chocolate Chip (Keebler)	1	80	4	11	0	75
Old-Fashion Chocolate Chip (Pepperidge Farm)	2	100	5	12	5	45
Old-Fashion Double Fudge (Keebler)	1	80	4	11	0	65
Old-Fashion Oatmeal (Keebler)	1	80	4	13	0	110
Old-Fashion Peanut Butter (Keebler)	1	80	4	10	0	100
Old-Fashion Sugar (Keebler)	1	80	3	13	0	70
Old-Time Molasses (Grandma's)	2 (2.75 oz)	320	9	58	5	520
Orange Milano (Pepperidge Farm)	2	150	7	17	5	60
Oreo (Nabisco)	1 (0.5 oz)	50	2	8	<2	75
Oreo, Double Stuf (Nabisco)	1 (0.5 oz)	70	4	9	<2	75
Oreo, Fudge Covered (Nabisco)	1 (0.75 oz)	110	6	13	<2	75

FOOD	PORTION	CAL	FAT	CARB	CHOL	SOD
Oreo Mini (Nabisco)	5 (0.5 oz)	70	3	10	0	85
Oreo, White Fudge Covered (Nabisco)	1 (0.75 oz)	110	6	14	<2	75
Orleans (Pepperidge Farm)	3	90	6	11	0	30
Orleans Sandwich (Pepperidge Farm)	2	120	8	14	0	40
Palmito (LU)	1	50	3	—	—	—
Paris (Pepperidge Farm)	2	100	5	—	—	—
Peach-Apricot Pastry, Dietetic (Stella D'Oro)	1	90	4	13	—	<10
Peanut Butter (Grandma's)	2 (2.75 oz)	410	30	43	10	410
Peanut Butter & Jelly Sandwiches (Little Debbie)	1 pkg (1.13 oz)	150	7	20	tr	105
Peanut Butter Bar (Frito Lay)	1.75 oz	270	16	30	0	65
Peanut Butter Bars (Little Debbie)	1 pkg (1.83 oz)	290	18	26	tr	180
Peanut Butter Creme Filled Wafer (Lance)	1 pkg (50 g)	240	10	34	0	80
Peanut Butter Naturals (Sunbelt)	1 pkg (1.2 oz)	170	10	19	—	90
Peanut Butter Sandwich (FFV)	2	170	8	—	—	—
Peanut Butter Wafers (Drake's)	1 (2.25 oz)	324	16	43	0	135
Peanut Clusters (Little Debbie)	1 pkg (1.44 oz)	210	11	25	tr	110
Pecan Crunch (Archway)	1	35	1	—	0	—
Pecan Shortbread (Pepperidge Farm)	1	70	5	7	0	15

FOOD	PORTION	CAL	FAT	CARB	CHOL	SOD
Pecan Supremes (Nabisco)	1 (0.5 oz)	80	5	9	<2	45
Pfeffernusse (Stella D'Oro)	1	40	1	7	tr	—
Pims (LU)	1	50	1	—	—	—
Pinwheels (Nabisco)	1 (1 oz)	130	5	20	0	35
Pirouettes, Chocolate Laced (Pepperidge Farm)	2	70	4	8	<5	20
Pirouettes, Original (Pepperidge Farm)	2	70	4	9	<5	35
Pitter Patter (Keebler)	1	90	4	12	0	115
Prune Pastry, Dietetic (Stella D'Oro)	1	90	4	13	—	<10
Pure Chocolate Middles (Nabisco)	1 (0.5 oz)	80	5	9	<5	35
Raisin Bran (Pepperidge Farm)	2	110	5	13	<5	55
Raisin Oatmeal (Archway)	1	35	1	—	0	—
Raisin, Soft (Grandma's)	2 (2.75 oz)	320	10	54	10	280
Raspberry Newtons (Nabisco)	1 (0.75 oz)	70	2	15	0	70
Regal Grahams (FFV)	2	140	7	—	—	—
Roman Egg Biscuits (Stella D'Oro)	1	140	5	20	tr	—
Royal Dainty (FFV)	2	120	6	—	—	—
Royal Nuggets (Stella D'Oro)	1	2	tr	tr	tr	—
Sandwich Cookies, Chocolate (Estee)	1	50	2	7	0	15
Sandwich Cookies, Original (Estee)	1	45	2	6	0	5

FOOD	PORTION	CAL	FAT	CARB	CHOL	SOD
Sandwich Cookies, Peanut Butter (Estee)	1	50	3	5	0	35
Sante Fe Oatmeal Raisin (Pepperidge Farm)	1	100	4	16	<5	70
Sausalito Milk Chocolate Macadamia (Pepperidge Farm)	1	120	7	14	5	65
Schoks-Chocolate (LU)	1	70	4	—	—	—
School House Cookies (Sunshine)	15	120	4	20	0	100
Sea Flappers (Sunshine)	7	140	6	20	0	80
Select Assortment (Archway)	1	60	2	—	5	—
Sesame Cookies (Stella D'Oro)	1	50	2	6	tr	—
Sesame Cookies Regina, Dietetic (Stella D'Oro)	1	40	2	6	—	<10
7-Grain Oatmeal (Frookie)	1	45	2	7	0	35
Seville (Pepperidge Farm)	2	100	5	—	—	—
Shortbread (Pepperidge Farm)	2	150	8	17	<5	85
Shortbread (Weight Watchers)	3	80	2	13	—	95
Snack Wafer, Chocolate (Estee)	1	80	4	11	0	—
Snack Wafer, Chocolate Coated (Estee)	1	130	7	14	0	10
Snack Wafer, Strawberry (Estee)	1	80	4	11	0	—

FOOD	PORTION	CAL	FAT	CARB	CHOL	SOD
Snack Wafer, Vanilla (Estee)	1	80	4	11	0	—
SnackWell's Chocolate Chip (Nabisco)	6 (0.5 oz)	60	1	11	0	85
SnackWell's Cinnamon Graham Snacks (Nabisco)	9 (0.5 oz)	50	0	12	0	50
SnackWell's Devil's Food Cakes (Nabisco)	1 (0.5 oz)	60	0	13	0	30
SnackWell's Oatmeal Raisin (Nabisco)	1 (0.5 oz)	60	1	10	0	65
Social Tea (Nabisco)	3 (0.5 oz)	70	2	11	<5	60
Soft 'n Chewy Chocolate Chip (Tastykake)	1 (39 g)	170	7	25	10	170
Soft 'n Chewy Chocolate Chocolate Chip (Tastykake)	1 (32 g)	170	7	26	5	110
Soft 'n Chewy Oatmeal Raisin (Tastykake)	1 (39 g)	160	5	27	5	160
Southport (Pepperidge Farm)	2	170	10	—	—	—
Sprinkles Rainbow Topping (Sunshine)	1	70	2	13	0	25
Strawberry Newtons (Nabisco)	1 (0.75 oz)	70	2	15	0	70
Sugar (Pepperidge Farm)	2	100	5	13	10	55
Sugar Wafers, Assorted (Sunshine)	2	90	4	12	<2	25
Sugar Wafers, Chocolate (Sunshine)	2	90	4	12	<2	15
Sugar Wafers, Peanut Butter (Sunshine)	2	80	4	10	<2	35

FOOD	PORTION	CAL	FAT	CARB	CHOL	SOD
Sugar Wafers, Vanilla (Sunshine)	2	90	4	12	<2	25
Swiss Fudge (Stella D'Oro)	1	70	3	9	tr	—
Taffy Creme Sandwich (Mother's)	1–2 (1 oz)	140	8	17	<2	80
Tahiti (Pepperidge Farm)	1	90	6	9	5	25
Tango (FFV)	2	160	5	—	—	—
T.C. Rounds (FFV)	2	160	8	—	—	—
Teddy Grahams Bearwich Chocolate & Vanilla Creme (Nabisco)	4 (0.5 oz)	70	3	10	0	60
Teddy Grahams Bearwich Chocolate Creme w/ Peanut Butter (Nabisco)	4 (0.5 oz)	70	3	10	0	65
Teddy Grahams Bearwich Cinnamon w/ Vanilla Creme (Nabisco)	4 (0.5 oz)	70	3	10	0	60
Teddy Grahams Bearwich Vanilla & Chocolate Creme (Nabisco)	4 (0.5 oz)	70	3	10	0	65
Teddy Grahams Chocolate Graham (Nal isco)	11 (0.5 oz)	60	2	10	0	90
Tedc y Grahams Cinnamon Graham (Nabisco)	11 (0.5 oz)	60	2	11	0	80
Teddy Grahams Honey Graham (Nabisco)	11 (0.5 oz)	60	2	11	0	90
Teddy Grahams Vanilla & Beach Bears (Nabisco)	11 (0.5 oz)	60	2	11	0	75

FOOD	PORTION	CAL	FAT	CARB	CHOL	SOD
Teddy Grahams Vanilla & Holiday Bears (Nabisco)	11 (0.5 oz)	60	2	11	0	75
Teddy Grahams Vanilla & Rockin' Bears (Nabisco)	11 (0.5 oz)	60	2	11	0	75
Teddy Grahams Vanilla Graham (Nabisco)	11 (0.5 oz)	60	2	10	0	75
The Great Tofu (Health Valley)	2	90	3	14	0	30
The Great Wheat Free (Health Valley)	2	80	3	14	0	35
Trolley Cakes Devilsfood (FFV)	2	120	2	—	—	—
Tru Blu Chocolate (Sunshine)	2	160	7	23	tr	140
Tru Blu Lemon (Sunshine)	1	70	3	12	tr	65
Tru Blu Vanilla (Sunshine)	1 (0.5 oz)	80	3	12	0	65
Vanilla Sugar Wafer (Tastykake)	1 (6 g)	36	2	4	0	10
Vanilla Wafers (FFV)	8	120	5	—	—	—
Vanilla Wafers (Keebler)	4	80	4	10	1	60
Vanilla Wafers (Sunshine)	3	70	3	9	<5	50
Van-O-Lunch (Lance)	1 pkg (37 g)	180	7	26	0	150
Vienna Fingers (Sunshine)	1 (0.5 oz)	70	3	10	0	60
Zurich (Pepperidge Farm)	1	60	2	10	0	30
animal crackers	1 (2.5 g)	11	tr	2	—	10
animal crackers	11 (1 oz)	126	4	21	—	112
animal crackers	1 box (2.4 oz)	299	9	51	11	274

FOOD	PORTION	CAL	FAT	CARB	CHOL	SOD
butter	1 (5 g)	23	1	3	—	18
chocolate chip	1 (0.4 oz)	48	2	7	—	32
chocolate chip	1 box (1.9 oz)	233	12	36	12	188
chocolate chip, low fat	1 (0.25 oz)	45	2	7	0	38
chocolate chip, low sugar & low sodium	1 (0.24 oz)	31	1	5	0	1
chocolate chip soft-type	1 (0.5 oz)	69	4	9	0	49
chocolate wafer	1 (0.2 oz)	26	1	1	0	35
chocolate wafer cookie crumbs	½ cup (5.9 oz)	728	25	120	0	980
chocolate w/ creme filling	1 (0.35 oz)	47	2	7	—	36
chocolate w/ creme filling, chocolate coated	1 (0.60 oz)	82	5	11	—	55
chocolate w/ creme filling, sugar free & low sodium	1 (0.35 oz)	46	2	7	—	24
chocolate w/ extra creme filling	1 (0.46 oz)	65	3	9	—	64
digestive biscuits, plain	2	141	7	21	—	—
fig bars	1 (0.56 oz)	56	1	11	—	56
fortune	1 (0.28 oz)	30	tr	7	—	22
fudge	1 (0.73 oz)	73	1	17	—	40
gingersnaps	1 (0.24 oz)	29	1	5	0	48
graham	1 sq (0.24 oz)	30	1	5	0	42
graham, chocolate covered	1 (0.49 oz)	68	3	9	0	41
graham cracker crumbs	½ cup (4.4 oz)	540	13	97	0	756
graham, honey	1 (0.24 oz)	30	1	5	0	42

FOOD	PORTION	CAL	FAT	CARB	CHOL	SOD
lady fingers	1 (0.38 oz)	40	1	7	40	16
marshmallow, chocolate coated	1 (0.46 oz)	55	2	9	—	22
marshmallow pie, chocolate coated	1 (1.4 oz)	165	7	26	—	66
molasses	1 (0.5 oz)	65	2	11	0	69
oatmeal	1 (0.6 oz)	81	3	12	0	69
oatmeal, soft-type	1 (0.5 oz)	61	2	10	—	52
oatmeal raisin	1 (0.6 oz)	81	3	12	0	69
oatmeal raisin, low sugar & no sodium	1 (0.24 oz)	31	1	5	0	1
oatmeat raisin, soft-type	1 (0.5 oz)	61	2	10	—	52
peanut butter, soft-type	1 (0.5 oz)	69	4	9	0	50
shortbread	1 (0.28 oz)	40	2	5	2	36
sugar	1 (0.52 oz)	72	3	10	8	53
sugar, low sugar & sodium free	1 (0.24 oz)	30	1	5	0	0
sugar wafers w/ creme filling	1 (0.12 oz)	18	1	3	0	5
sugar wafers w/ creme filling, sugar free & sodium free	1 (0.14 oz)	20	1	3	0	0
vanilla sandwich	1 (0.35 oz)	48	2	7	0	35
vanilla wafers	1 (0.21 oz)	28	1	4	—	18

DOUGHNUTS

FOOD	PORTION	CAL	FAT	CARB	CHOL	SOD
Cinnamon (Tastykake)	1 (47 g)	180	8	26	10	210
Cinnamon Apple (Earth Grains)	1	310	17	—	25	—
Crumb Topped (Entenmann's)	1 (2.1 oz)	260	12	34	—	220

FOOD	PORTION	CAL	FAT	CARB	CHOL	SOD
Devil's Food (Earth Grains)	1	330	21	—	20	—
Devil's Food Crumb (Entenmann's)	1 (2.1 oz)	250	12	34	—	200
Donut Sticks (Little Debbie)	1 pkg (1.67 oz)	200	9	29	tr	220
Frosted Rich (Tastykake)	1 (57 g)	260	16	28	10	200
Frosted Rich Mini (Tastykake)	1 (14 g)	44	3	8	5	60
Glazed Old Fashioned (Earth Grains)	1	310	18	—	20	—
Honey Wheat (Tastykake)	1 (57 g)	210	8	32	10	200
Honey Wheat Mini (Tastykake)	1 (12 g)	40	1	7	5	50
Old-Fashion Donuts (Drake's)	1 (1.7 oz)	182	8	25	10	238
Orange Glazed (Tastykake)	1 (57 g)	210	9	32	10	180
Plain (Dutch Mill)	1 (1.75 oz)	220	10	22	—	—
Plain (Tastykake)	1 (47 g)	190	10	—	10	170
Powdered Old Fashioned (Earth Grains)	1	290	19	—	20	—
Powdered Sugar (Tastykake)	1 (46 g)	180	9	24	24	220
Powdered Sugar Donut Delites (Drake's)	7 (2.5 oz)	300	15	38	16	316
Powdered Sugar Mini (Tastykake)	1 (12 g)	40	1	7	5	70
Rich Frosted (Entenmann's)	1 (2 oz)	280	18	27	—	210
cake type, unsugared	1 (1.6 oz)	198	11	23	18	257

FOOD	PORTION	CAL	FAT	CARB	CHOL	SOD
chocolate coated	1 (1.5 oz)	204	13	21	—	185
chocolate glazed	1 (1.5 oz)	175	8	24	—	143
chocolate sugared	1 (1.5 oz)	175	8	24	—	143
creme filled	1 (3 oz)	307	21	26	20	262
french cruller, glazed	1 (1.4 oz)	169	8	24	5	142
frosted	1 (1.5 oz)	204	13	21	—	185
honey bun	1 (2.1 oz)	242	14	27	4	205
jelly	1 (3 oz)	289	16	33	22	249
old fashioned	1 (1.6 oz)	198	11	23	18	257
sugared	1 (1.6 oz)	192	10	23	14	181
wheat, glazed	1 (1.6 oz)	162	9	19	9	160
wheat, sugared	1 (1.6 oz)	162	9	19	9	160
yeast, glazed	1 (2.1 oz)	242	14	26	4	205

ICE CREAM AND FROZEN DESSERTS

FOOD	PORTION	CAL	FAT	CARB	CHOL	SOD
All Flavors Avari Creme Glacé	1 oz	10	0	3	0	35
All Flavors Royale Cremes (Bresler's)	4 oz	260	16	24	48	—
All Flavors Royale Lites (Bresler's)	4 oz	217	0	49	0	—
All Flavors Ice Cream (Bresler's)	3.5 oz	230	12	23	36	—
Almond Praline Light (Edy's)	4 oz	140	5	18	15	50
Banana Cream (Fi-Bar)	1 bar	93	tr	21	—	—
Banana-Politan Light (Edy's)	4 oz	110	4	15	15	50
Berry Berry Berry (Mocha Mix)	3.5 oz	209	9	30	0	99
Berry Swirl Bar, Raspberry (Carnation)	1 bar	70	3	—	10	—

FOOD	PORTION	CAL	FAT	CARB	CHOL	SOD
Berry Swirl Bar, Strawberry (Carnation)	1 bar	70	3	—	9	—
Black Cherry Fat Free (Borden)	½ cup	90	tr	21	0	40
Black Cherry Free (Sealtest)	½ cup	100	0	25	0	45
Bordeaux Cherry (Healthy Choice)	4 oz	120	1	23	5	50
Bounty Cherry, Dark (M&M's)	1 (0.84 fl oz)	70	5	8	5	20
Bounty Coconut, Dark (M&M's)	1 (0.84 fl oz)	70	5	7	5	20
Bounty Coconut, Milk (M&M's)	1 (0.84 fl oz)	70	5	7	5	20
Bubble Crazy (Good Humor)	3 oz	74	1	—	—	—
Bubble O Bill (Good Humor)	3.5 oz	149	8	—	—	—
Butter Almond (Breyers)	½ cup	170	10	15	25	125
Butter Crunch (Sealtest)	½ cup	150	7	18	25	90
Butter Pecan (Breyers)	½ cup	180	12	15	25	125
Butter Pecan (Frusen Gladje)	½ cup	280	21	16	60	160
Butter Pecan (Haagen-Dazs)	4 oz	390	24	29	115	100
Butter Pecan (Sealtest)	½ cup	160	9	16	15	125
Butter Pecan Light (Edy's)	4 oz	140	5	18	15	50
Buttered Pecan (Borden)	½ cup	180	12	16	—	65

FOOD	PORTION	CAL	FAT	CARB	CHOL	SOD
Cafe Au Lait Light (Edy's)	4 oz	110	4	13	15	50
Candy Bar Light (Edy's)	4 oz	140	5	20	15	50
Cappuccino (Rice Dream)	½ cup	130	5	17	0	80
Caramel Almond Crunch Bar (Haagen-Dazs)	1	240	18	17	40	65
Caramel Nut Ice Milk (Light N' Lively)	½ cup	120	4	18	10	85
Caramel Nut Sundae (Haagen-Dazs)	4 oz	310	21	26	—	100
Carob (Rice Dream)	½ cup	130	5	20	0	80
Carob (Tofu Ice Creme)	4 fl oz	190	8	28	0	55
Carob Almond (Rice Dream)	½ cup	140	6	20	0	80
Carob Chip (Rice Dream)	½ cup	140	6	20	0	80
Carob Chip Mint (Rice Dream)	½ cup	140	6	20	0	80
Cheesecake Bar, Original (Carnation)	1 bar	120	6	—	12	—
Cheesecake Bar, Strawberry (Carnation)	1 bar	125	6	—	10	—
Cherry & Ice Cream Swirl (Chiquita)	1 bar	80	3	—	—	—
Cherry Cola Kick (Good Humor)	4.5 oz	106	1	—	—	—
Cherry Garcia (Ben & Jerry's)	½ cup	230	16	23	80	35
Cherry Garcia (Ben & Jerry's)	1 pop (3.7 fl oz)	250	18	25	45	100

FOOD	PORTION	CAL	FAT	CARB	CHOL	SOD
Cherry Vanilla (Breyers)	½ cup	150	7	17	20	45
Chip Candy Crunch (Good Humor)	3 oz	347	24	—	—	—
Chocolate (Ben & Jerry's)	½ cup	230	14	24	55	25
Chocolate (Breyers)	½ cup	160	8	20	20	30
Chocolate (Frusen Gladje)	½ cup	240	17	17	75	65
Chocolate (Haagen-Dazs)	4 oz	270	17	24	120	50
Chocolate (Healthy Choice)	4 oz	130	2	24	5	70
Chocolate (Sealtest)	½ cup	140	6	18	20	50
Chocolate (Simple Pleasures)	4 oz	140	tr	25	10	—
Chocolate (Ultra Slim-Fast)	4 oz	100	tr	19	0	45
Chocolate American Dream (Edy's)	3 oz	90	1	20	0	45
Chocolate Bar (Rice Dream)	1	270	16	33	0	115
Chocolate Caramel Sundae Light (Simple Pleasures)	4 oz	90	tr	20	15	—
Chocolate Chip (Sealtest)	½ cup	150	8	17	15	50
Chocolate Chip (Simple Pleasures)	4 oz	150	3	25	15	—
Chocolate Chip American Dream (Edy's)	3 oz	100	1	22	0	45
Chocolate Chip Cookie Dough (Ben & Jerry's)	1 pop (2.5 fl oz)	240	16	26	45	110

FOOD	PORTION	CAL	FAT	CARB	CHOL	SOD
Chocolate Chip Cookie Dough (Ben & Jerry's)	½ cup	260	17	29	85	65
Chocolate Chip Ice Milk (Weight Watchers)	½ cup	120	4	18	10	80
Chocolate Chip Ice Milk (Light N' Lively)	½ cup	120	4	18	10	35
Chocolate Chip Light (Edy's)	4 oz	120	4	16	15	50
Chocolate Chocolate Chip (Frusen Gladje)	½ cup	270	18	21	55	60
Chocolate Chocolate Chip (Haagen-Dazs)	4 oz	290	20	28	105	40
Chocolate Chocolate Mint (Haagen-Dazs)	4 oz	300	20	26	—	50
Chocolate Coated Vanilla Ice Cream (Good Humor)	3 oz	198	14	—	—	—
Chocolate Dark Chocolate Bar (Haagen-Dazs)	1	390	27	32	—	60
Chocolate Dip Bar (Weight Watchers)	1 (2 oz)	110	7	10	5	45
Chocolate Eclair (Good Humor)	3 oz	187	10	—	—	—
Chocolate Fat Free (Borden)	½ cup	100	tr	21	0	50
Chocolate Fat-Free Frozen Dessert (Weight Watchers)	½ cup	80	0	19	5	75
Chocolate Free (Sealtest)	½ cup	100	0	23	0	50
Chocolate Fudge (Ultra Slim-Fast)	4 oz	120	tr	24	0	65

FOOD	PORTION	CAL	FAT	CARB	CHOL	SOD
Chocolate Fudge Brownie (Ben & Jerry's)	½ cup	250	14	29	50	85
Chocolate Fudge Cake (Good Humor)	6.3 oz	214	15	—	—	—
Chocolate Fudge Mousse Light (Edy's)	4 oz	130	5	18	15	50
Chocolate Fudge Swirl Dessert Bar Free (Sealtest)	1	90	0	19	0	30
Chocolate Fudge Twirl Ice Milk Light (Breyers)	½ cup	130	4	21	10	60
Chocolate Ice Milk (Borden)	½ cup	100	2	18	—	80
Chocolate Ice Milk Light (Breyers)	½ cup	120	4	18	15	55
Chocolate Light (Simple Pleasures)	4 oz	80	tr	16	15	—
Chocolate Malt (Good Humor)	3 oz	187	13	—	—	—
Chocolate Malted Bars (Carnation)	1 bar	70	3	—	19	—
Chocolate Marshmallow Sundae (Sealtest)	½ cup	150	6	21	20	40
Chocolate Mousse Bar, Sugar Free (Weight Watchers)	1 (1.75 oz)	35	tr	9	5	30
Chocolate Nutty Bar (Rice Dream)	1	330	23	29	0	110
Chocolate Peanut Butter Chocolate Chip Cookie Dough (Ben & Jerry's)	½ cup	280	18	28	55	60
Chocolate Swirl (Borden)	½ cup	130	6	18	—	65

FOOD	PORTION	CAL	FAT	CARB	CHOL	SOD
Chocolate Swirl Fat-Free Frozen Dessert (Weight Watchers)	½ cup	90	0	22	5	75
Chocolate Treat Bar, Sugar Free (Weight Watchers)	1 (2.75 oz)	90	0	18	0	75
Chunky Monkey (Ben & Jerry's)	½ cup	270	19	27	70	25
Cocoa-Fudge 'N Cream (Fi-Bar)	1 bar	93	tr	21	—	—
Cocoa Marble Fudge (Rice Dream)	½ cup	140	6	19	0	80
Coconut Bar (Good Humor)	3 oz	207	14	—	—	—
Coffee (Breyers)	½ cup	150	8	16	30	50
Coffee (Haagen-Dazs)	4 oz	270	17	23	120	55
Coffee (Sealtest)	½ cup	140	7	16	15	50
Coffee (Simple Pleasures)	4 oz	120	tr	22	15	—
Coffee Heath Bar Crunch (Ben & Jerry's)	½ cup	270	19	26	80	100
Coffee Ice Milk (Light N' Lively)	½ cup	100	3	16	10	40
Combo Cup, Vanilla/Chocolate (Good Humor)	6 oz	201	9	—	—	—
Cookies n' Cream (Breyers)	½ cup	170	9	19	70	60
Cookies N' Cream (Healthy Choice)	4 oz	130	2	24	5	80
Cookies n' Cream (Simple Pleasures)	4 oz	150	2	25	5	—
Cookies 'N' Cream American Dream (Edy's)	3 oz	100	1	22	0	45

FOOD	PORTION	CAL	FAT	CARB	CHOL	SOD
Cookies n'Cream Ice Milk (Light N' Lively)	½ cup	110	3	18	10	65
Cookies 'N' Cream Light (Edy's)	4 oz	120	5	18	15	50
Cool 'N Creamy Amaretto w/ Chocolate Swirl	1 bar	62	2	10	1	50
Cool 'N Creamy Chocolate/Vanilla	1 bar	54	2	7	1	51
Cool 'N Creamy Double Chocolate Fudge	1 bar	55	2	7	1	57
Cool 'N Creamy Orange/Vanilla	1 bar	31	1	5	tr	18
Creamy Lites Bar, Chocolate (Carnation)	1 bar	50	2	—	8	—
Creamy Lites Bar, Strawberry (Carnation)	1 bar	50	2	—	7	—
Deep Chocolate (Haagen-Dazs)	4 oz	290	14	26	—	70
Deep Chocolate Fudge (Haagen-Dazs)	4 oz	290	14	26	—	90
Deluxe Sundae (Good Humor)	6 oz	300	11	—	—	—
Double Fudge Bar (Weight Watchers)	1 (1.75 oz)	60	1	12	5	50
DoveBar, Almond (M&M's)	1 (3.67 fl oz)	335	22	30	35	75
DoveBar, Caramel Pecan (M&M's)	1 (3.67 fl oz)	350	35	35	35	85
DoveBar, Chocolate w/ Milk Chocolate (M&M's)	1 (3.8 fl oz)	340	21	35	40	80
DoveBar, Coffee Cashew (M&M's)	1 (3.67 fl oz)	335	22	31	35	55

FOOD	PORTION	CAL	FAT	CARB	CHOL	SOD
DoveBar, Crunchy Cookie (M&M's)	1 (3.8 fl oz)	340	21	35	40	65
DoveBar, Peanut (M&M's)	1 (3.8 fl oz)	380	25	35	40	100
DoveBar, Vanilla w/ Dark Chocolate (M&M's)	1 (3.8 fl oz)	340	22	34	45	65
Dovebar, Vanilla w/ Milk Chocolate (M&M's)	1 (3.8 fl oz)	340	21	34	40	60
Dove Bite-Size Almond Praline (M&M's)	1 (0.75 fl oz)	80	5	8	7	15
Dove Bite-Size Cherry Royale (M&M's)	1 (0.75 fl oz)	70	5	8	8	10
Dove Bite-Size Classic Vanilla (M&M's)	1 (0.75 fl oz)	70	5	7	8	10
Dove Bite-Size French Vanilla (M&M's)	1 (0.75 fl oz)	70	5	7	15	10
Dove Bite-Size Mint Supreme (M&M's)	1 (0.75 fl oz)	80	5	8	7	5
Dream Pie, Chocolate (Rice Dream)	1	380	19	47	0	225
Dream Pie, Mint (Rice Dream)	1	380	19	47	0	225
Dream Pie, Mocha (Rice Dream)	1	380	19	47	0	225
Dream Pie, Vanilla (Rice Dream)	1	380	19	47	0	225
Dreamy Caramel Cream Light (Edy's)	4 oz	140	4	16	15	50
Dutch Chocolate (Mocha Mix)	3.5 oz	210	12	25	0	135
Dutch Chocolate Olde-Fashioned Recipe (Borden)	½ cup	130	6	16	—	65

FOOD	PORTION	CAL	FAT	CARB	CHOL	SOD
English Toffee Crunch Bar (Weight Watchers)	1 (2 oz)	120	11	11	5	60
Fat Frog (Good Humor)	3 oz	154	9	—	—	—
Finger Bar, Strawberry (Good Humor)	2.5 oz	49	tr	—	0	—
Fosters Freeze, Vanilla	1 oz	43	1	—	—	—
French Vanilla (Sealtest)	½ cup	140	7	16	35	50
Fresh Lites, Chocolate Chip (Dole)	1 bar	60	1	10	—	30
Fudge Bar (Good Humor)	2.5 oz	127	tr	—	—	—
Fudge Bar (Ultra Slim-Fast)	1	90	tr	17	0	50
Fudge Pop Bar (Haagen-Dazs)	1	210	14	19	—	50
Fudge Royale (Sealtest)	½ cup	140	7	19	15	55
Full O'Chocolate (Good Humor)	3 oz	245	18	—	—	—
Gummy Dinosaur Colossal Fossil Lemon/Cherry (Good Humor)	3 oz	75	tr	—	0	—
Gummy Dinosaur Colossal Fossil Lemon/Grape (Good Humor)	3 oz	75	tr	—	0	—
Heath Bar Crunch (Ben & Jerry's)	½ cup	270	19	26	85	100
Heath Bar Crunch (Ben & Jerry's)	1 pop (3.7 fl oz)	340	23	35	50	90

FOOD	PORTION	CAL	FAT	CARB	CHOL	SOD
Heath Bar Crunch (Ben & Jerry's)	1 pop (2.5 fl oz)	260	18	25	35	65
Heaven Bars, Vanilla Caramel Nut (Carnation)	1 bar	225	15	—	9	—
Heaven Bars, Vanilla Nut Fudge (Carnation)	1 bar	222	15	—	9	—
Heaven Sundae Bars, Chocolate Fudge (Carnation)	1 bar	150	9	—	7	—
Heaven Sundae Bars, Vanilla Fudge (Carnation)	1 bar	150	9	—	7	—
Heavenly Hash (Mocha Mix)	3.5 oz	244	13	29	0	116
Heavenly Hash (Sealtest)	½ cup	150	7	19	15	50
Heavenly Hash Ice Milk (Light N' Lively)	½ cup	120	4	20	10	35
Heavenly Hash Ice Milk Light (Breyers)	½ cup	150	5	21	10	55
Honey Vanilla (Haagen-Dazs)	4 oz	250	16	22	135	55
Ice Cream Sandwich, Chocolate w/ Chocolate Chip Cookie (Good Humor)	4 oz	268	11	—	—	—
Ice Cream Sandwich, Vanilla w/ Chocolate Chip Cookie (Good Humor)	4 oz	246	11	—	—	—
Ice Cream Sandwich, Vanilla (Good Humor)	2.5 oz	162	5	—	—	—
Jumbo Jet Star (Good Humor)	4.5 oz	85	tr	—	—	—
King Cone (Good Humor)	5.5 oz	315	19	—	—	—

FOOD	PORTION	CAL	FAT	CARB	CHOL	SOD
Lemon (Rice Dream)	½ cup	130	5	17	0	80
Macadamia Brittle (Haagen-Dazs)	4 oz	280	18	25	—	60
Malt Ball 'N' Fudge Light (Edy's)	4 oz	140	5	20	15	50
Maple Walnut (Sealtest)	½ cup	160	9	17	20	40
Marble Fudge Light (Edy's)	4 oz	120	4	15	15	50
Mars Almond Bar (M&M's)	1 (1.85 fl oz)	210	14	20	15	45
Milk Chocolate Almond (Ben & Jerry's)	1 pop (2.5 fl oz)	250	19	16	35	85
Milky Way Single, Chocolate w/ milk Chocolate (M&M's)	1 (2 fl oz)	210	11	24	20	60
Milky Way Single, Vanilla w/ Dark Chocolate (M&M's)	1 (2 fl oz)	200	12	24	20	50
Milky Way Snack, Chocolate w/ Milk Chocolate (M&M's)	1 (0.72 fl oz)	70	4	9	5	25
Milky Way Snack, Vanilla w/ Dark Chocolate (M&M's)	1 (0.72 fl oz)	70	4	9	5	25
Mint Chocolate (Breyers)	½ cup	170	10	18	45	45
Mint Chocolate Chocolate Chip (Simple Pleasures)	4 oz	150	2	26	5	—
Mint Cookie (Ben & Jerry's)	½ cup	250	17	25	85	100
Mixed Berry & Ice Cream Swirl (Chiquita)	1 bar	80	3	—	—	—

FOOD	PORTION	CAL	FAT	CARB	CHOL	SOD
Mocha Almond Fudge (Mocha Mix)	3.5 oz	229	11	29	0	113
Mocha Almond Fudge American Dream (Edy's)	3 oz	110	1	24	0	45
Mocha Almond Fudge Light (Edy's)	4 oz	140	5	19	15	50
Neapolitan (Healthy Choice)	4 oz	120	2	26	5	60
Neapolitan (Mocha Mix)	3.5 oz	208	11	22	0	120
Neapolitan Fat Free Frozen Dessert (Weight Watchers)	½ cup	80	0	19	5	75
New York Super Fudge (Ben & Jerry's)	1 pop (2.5 fl oz)	330	26	22	25	125
New York Super Fudge (Ben & Jerry's)	1 pop (3.7 fl oz)	330	26	22	25	135
New York Super Fudge (Ben & Jerry's)	½ cup	290	20	26	45	40
ONE-ders Brownies 'n Creme (Weight Watchers)	4 oz	130	4	20	10	115
ONE-ders Chocolate Chip (Weight Watchers)	4 oz	120	4	18	10	80
ONE-ders Heavenly Hash (Weight Watchers)	4 oz	130	3	22	10	90
ONE-ders Pralines 'n Creme (Weight Watchers)	4 oz	130	4	19	10	90
ONE-ders Strawberry (Weight Watchers)	4 oz	110	3	17	10	75

FOOD	PORTION	CAL	FAT	CARB	CHOL	SOD
Orange & Cream Pop (Haagen-Dazs)	1	130	6	18	—	25
Orange & Ice Cream Swirl (Chiquita)	1 bar	80	3	—	—	—
Orange Vanilla Treat Bar, Sugar Free & Fat Free (Weight Watchers)	1 (1.75 oz)	30	0	9	0	40
Peach (Breyers)	½ cup	130	6	18	15	35
Peach (Mocha Mix)	3.5 oz	198	9	28	0	96
Peach (Simple Pleasures)	4 oz	120	tr	21	10	—
Peach (Ultra Slim-Fast)	4 oz	100	tr	22	0	55
Peach, Fat Free (Borden)	½ cup	90	tr	21	0	40
Peach Free (Sealtest)	½ cup	100	0	23	0	45
Peanut Butter & Chocolate Light (Edy's)	4 oz	130	5	19	15	50
Peanut Butter Crunch Bar (Haagen-Dazs)	1	270	21	16	35	55
Peanut Butter Fudge (Rice Dream)	½ cup	160	7	19	0	100
Peanut Fudge Sundae (Sealtest)	½ cup	140	7	17	20	50
Pecan Praline (Simple Pleasures)	4 oz	140	2	25	5	—
Pecan Pralines 'n Creme Ice Milk (Weight Watchers)	½ cup	130	4	20	10	90
Praline Almond Ice Milk Light (Breyers)	½ cup	130	5	19	10	70
Praline & Caramel (Healthy Choice)	4 oz	130	2	26	5	70

FOOD	PORTION	CAL	FAT	CARB	CHOL	SOD
Pralines & Caramel (Ultra Slim-Fast)	4 oz	120	tr	25	0	95
Rain Forest Crunch (Ben & Jerry's)	½ cup	270	21	21	85	100
Rain Forest Crunch (Ben & Jerry's)	1 pop (3.7 fl oz)	350	27	26	50	195
Raspberries 'N Cream (Fi-Bar)	1 bar	93	tr	21	—	—
Raspberry Truffle Light (Edy's)	4 oz	110	5	19	15	50
Raspberry & Ice Cream Swirl (Chiquita)	1 bar	80	3	—	—	—
Rocky Road (Healthy Choice)	4 oz	140	1	29	5	70
Rocky Road American Dream (Edy's)	3 oz	110	1	24	0	45
Rocky Road Light (Edy's)	4 oz	130	5	17	15	50
Rum Raisin (Haagen-Dazs)	4 oz	250	17	21	110	45
Rum Raisin (Simple Pleasures)	4 oz	130	tr	35	15	—
Scribbler (Good Humor)	3 oz	120	1	—	—	—
Shark Bar (Good Humor)	3 oz	63	tr	—	—	—
Snickers Single (M&M's)	1 (2 fl oz)	220	13	22	15	65
Snickers Snack (M&M's)	1 (1 fl oz)	110	7	11	5	35
Strawberries and Cream (Good Humor)	3 oz	96	2	—	—	—
Strawberries 'N Cream Olde-Fashioned Recipe (Borden)	½ cup	130	5	19	—	55

FOOD	PORTION	CAL	FAT	CARB	CHOL	SOD
Strawberry (Borden)	½ cup	130	6	18	—	55
Strawberry (Breyers)	½ cup	130	6	16	20	40
Strawberry (Frusen Gladje)	½ cup	230	15	20	65	60
Strawberry (Haagen-Dazs)	4 oz	250	15	23	95	40
Strawberry (Healthy Choice)	4 oz	110	1	21	5	50
Strawberry (Rice Dream)	½ cup	130	5	17	0	80
Strawberry (Sealtest)	½ cup	130	5	18	15	40
Strawberry (Simple Pleasures)	4 oz	120	tr	22	10	—
Strawberry American Dream (Edy's)	3 oz	70	tr	16	0	40
Strawberry & Ice Cream Swirl (Chiquita)	1 bar	80	3	—	—	—
Strawberry Bar (Rice Dream)	1	260	15	31	0	110
Strawberry Fat Free (Borden)	½ cup	90	tr	21	0	40
Strawberry Free (Sealtest)	½ cup	100	0	23	0	40
Strawberry Ice Milk (Borden)	½ cup	90	2	17	—	65
Strawberry Ice Milk Light (Breyers)	½ cup	110	3	18	15	50
Strawberry Light (Edy's)	4 oz	110	4	15	15	50
Strawberry Shortcake (Good Humor)	3 oz	186	12	—	—	—
Strawberry Swirl (Mocha Mix)	3.5 oz	209	9	30	0	98
Sundae Cone (Borden)	1	210	12	23	—	110

FOOD	PORTION	CAL	FAT	CARB	CHOL	SOD
Sundae Cone (Meadow Gold)	1	210	12	23	—	110
Supreme (Good Humor)	3.5 oz	342	23	—	—	—
Swiss Chocolate Candy Almond (Frusen Gladje)	½ cup	270	19	18	55	60
3 Musketeers Single, Chocolate (M&M's)	1 (2 fl oz)	160	10	16	20	30
3 Musketeers Single, Vanilla (M&M's)	1 (2 fl oz)	160	10	16	15	30
3 Musketeers Snack, Chocolate (M&M's)	1 (0.72 fl oz)	60	4	6	5	10
3 Musketeers Snack, Vanilla (M&M's)	1 (0.72 fl oz)	60	4	6	5	10
Toasted Almond (Good Humor)	3 oz	193	10	—	—	—
Toasted Almond (Mocha Mix)	3.5 oz	229	13	26	0	117
Toasted Almond American Dream (Edy's)	3 oz	110	1	24	0	45
Toffee Crunch (Simple Pleasures)	4 oz	130	tr	22	10	—
Toffee Fudge Parfait Ice Milk Light (Breyers)	½ cup	140	5	22	10	90
Tofulite	4 oz	150	7	—	0	—
Tofutti						
Cappuccino Love Drops	4 oz	230	12	—	0	—
Chocolate Cuties	4 oz	140	5	—	0	—
Chocolate Love Drops	4 oz	220	13	—	0	—
Chocolate Supreme	4 oz	210	13	—	0	—

FOOD	PORTION	CAL	FAT	CARB	CHOL	SOD
Lite lite Applejack Vanilla Twirl	4 oz	90	tr	—	0	—
Lite lite Cappuccino Vanilla Twirl	4 oz	90	tr	—	0	—
Lite lite Chocolate Strawberry Twirl	4 oz	90	tr	—	0	—
Lite lite Chocolate Vanilla Twirl	4 oz	90	tr	—	0	—
Lite lite Strawberry Vanilla Twirl	4 oz	90	tr	—	0	—
Lite lite Vanilla/ Chocolate/ Strawberry Twirl	4 oz	90	tr	—	0	—
Soft Serve Hi-Lite Chocolate	4 oz	100	1	—	0	—
Soft Serve Hi-Lite Vanilla	4 oz	90	1	—	0	—
Soft Serve Regular	4 oz	158	8	—	0	—
Vanilla	4 oz	200	11	—	0	—
Vanilla Almond Bark	4 oz	230	14	—	0	—
Vanilla Cuties	4 oz	130	5	—	0	—
Vanilla Love Drops	4 oz	220	12	—	0	—
Wildberry	4 oz	210	12	—	0	—
Triple Chocolate Stripes (Sealtest)	½ cup	140	7	17	20	50
Twister (Good Humor)	3 oz	131	7	—	—	—
Vanilla (Ben & Jerry's)	½ cup	215	16	18	95	30
Vanilla (Breyer's)	½ cup	150	8	15	25	50
Vanilla (Eagle Brand)	½ cup	150	9	16	—	55
Vanilla (Frusen Gladje)	½ cup	230	17	16	65	70

FOOD	PORTION	CAL	FAT	CARB	CHOL	SOD
Vanilla (Haagen-Dazs)	4 oz	260	17	23	120	55
Vanilla (Healthy Choice)	4 oz	120	2	21	5	60
Vanilla (Land O'Lakes)	4 oz	140	7	—	30	—
Vanilla (Mocha Mix)	3.5 oz	209	11	26	0	117
Vanilla (Rice Dream)	½ cup	130	5	17	0	80
Vanilla (Sealtest)	½ cup	140	7	16	20	50
Vanilla (Simple Pleasures)	4 oz	120	tr	22	15	—
Vanilla (Tofu Ice Cream)	4 fl oz	190	8	28	0	55
Vanilla (Ultra Slim-Fast)	4 oz	90	tr	19	0	55
Vanilla American Dream (Edy's)	3 oz	80	tr	18	0	45
Vanilla Bar (Rice Dream)	1	275	16	33	0	120
Vanilla Brownie (Ben & Jerry's)	1 bar	260	14	32	50	165
Vanilla Chocolate Chunk (Ben & Jerry's)	½ cup	250	18	24	85	30
Vanilla Chocolate Sandwich (Ultra Slim-Fast)	1	140	2	28	0	220
Vanilla, Chocolate, Strawberry (Edy's)	4 oz	110	4	14	15	50
Vanilla, Chocolate, Strawberry American Dream (Edy's)	3 oz	80	1	18	0	45
Vanilla Cookie Crunch Bar (Ultra Slim-Fast)	1	90	4	14	0	70
Vanilla Crunch Bar (Haagen-Dazs)	1	220	16	16	40	55

FOOD	PORTION	CAL	FAT	CARB	CHOL	SOD
Vanilla Cup (Good Humor)	3 oz	98	5	—	—	—
Vanilla Fat Free (Borden)	½ cup	90	tr	20	0	50
Vanilla Fat Free Frozen Dessert (Weight Watchers)	½ cup	80	0	20	5	75
Vanilla Free (Sealtest)	½ cup	100	0	24	0	45
Vanilla Fudge (Haagen-Dazs)	4 oz	270	17	26	—	—
Vanilla Fudge (Rice Dream)	½ cup	140	6	21	0	80
Vanilla Fudge Cookie (Ultra Slim-Fast)	4 oz	110	tr	24	0	90
Vanilla Fudge Royale Free (Sealtest)	½ cup	100	0	24	0	50
Vanilla Fudge Swirl Dessert Bar Free (Sealtest)	1	80	0	18	0	30
Vanilla Fudge Swirl Light (Simple Pleasures)	4 oz	90	tr	20	15	—
Vanilla Fudge Twirl (Breyers)	½ cup	160	8	19	20	55
Vanilla Fudge Twirl Ice Milk (Light N' Lively)	½ cup	110	3	18	10	45
Vanilla Ice Milk (Borden)	½ cup	90	2	17	—	65
Vanilla Ice Milk (Land O'Lakes)	4 oz	90	3	—	10	—
Vanilla Ice Milk (Light N' Lively)	½ cup	100	3	16	10	40
Vanilla Ice Milk Light (Breyer's)	½ cup	120	4	18	10	60
Vanilla Light (Edy's)	4 oz	100	4	13	15	50

FOOD	PORTION	CAL	FAT	CARB	CHOL	SOD
Vanilla Light (Simple Pleasures)	4 oz	80	tr	16	15	—
Vanilla Milk Chocolate Almond Bar (Haagen-Dazs)	1	370	27	27	—	55
Vanilla Milk Chocolate Bar (Haagen-Dazs)	1	360	27	26	—	55
Vanilla Milk Chocolate Brittle Bar (Haagen-Dazs)	1	370	25	32	—	160
Vanilla Nutty Bar (Rice Dream)	1	330	23	29	0	100
Vanilla Oatmeal Sandwich (Ultra Slim-Fast)	1	150	3	26	0	160
Vanilla Old Fashioned (Healthy Choice)	4 oz	120	2	21	5	60
Vanilla Olde-Fashioned Recipe (Borden)	½ cup	130	7	15	—	55
Vanilla Peanut Butter Swirl (Haagen-Dazs)	4 oz	280	21	19	110	120
Vanilla Red Raspberry Parfait Ice Milk Light (Breyers)	½ cup	130	3	23	15	50
Vanilla Sandwich (Ultra Slim-Fast)	1	140	2	28	0	220
Vanilla Sandwich Bar, Fat Free (Weight Watchers)	1 (2.5 oz)	130	0	30	—	170
Vanilla Strawberry Royale Free (Sealtest)	½ cup	100	0	25	0	35
Vanilla Strawberry Swirl Dessert Bar Free (Sealtest)	1	80	0	17	0	40
Vanilla Swiss Almond (Haagen-Dazs)	4 oz	290	19	24	—	55

FOOD	PORTION	CAL	FAT	CARB	CHOL	SOD
Vanilla Swiss Almond (Frusen Gladje)	½ cup	270	19	18	60	65
Vanilla Swiss Almond (Rice Dream)	½ cup	140	6	20	0	80
Vanilla w/ Chocolate Covered Almonds Ice Milk (Light N' Lively)	½ cup	120	4	17	10	45
Vanilla w/ Orange Sherbet (Sealtest)	½ cup	130	4	22	15	40
Vanilla w/ Red Raspberry Sherbet (Sealtest)	½ cup	130	4	22	15	40
Vanilla w/ Raspberry Twirl Ice Milk (Light N' Lively)	½ cup	110	3	19	10	35
Viennetta Petites, Chocolate Mint (Good Humor)	5 oz	236	14	—	—	—
Viennetta Petites, Vanilla (Good Humor)	5 oz	236	14	—	—	—
Viennetta Regular, Chocolate (Good Humor)	5 oz	225	14	—	—	—
Viennetta Regular, Vanilla (Good Humor)	5 oz	225	14	—	—	—
Whammy (Good Humor)	1.6 oz	95	7	—	—	—
Wildberry (Rice Dream)	½ cup	130	5	17	0	80
Wild Berry Swirl (Healthy Choice)	4 oz	120	2	23	5	60
cone, vanilla ice milk soft serve	1 (4.6 oz)	164	6	24	28	92
french vanilla soft serve	1 cup	377	23	38	153	153
french vanilla soft serve	½ gal	3014	180	306	1226	1228

FOOD	PORTION	CAL	FAT	CARB	CHOL	SOD
sundae, caramel	1 (5.4 oz)	303	9	49	25	195
sundae, hot fudge	1 (5.4 oz)	284	9	48	21	182
sundae, strawberry	1 (5.4 oz)	269	8	45	21	92
vanilla, 10% fat	1 cup	269	14	32	59	116
vanilla, 10% fat	½ gal	2153	115	254	476	929
vanilla, 16% fat	1 cup	349	24	32	88	108
vanilla, 16% fat	½ gal	2805	190	256	256	868
vanilla ice milk	1 cup	184	6	29	18	105
vanilla ice milk	½ gal	1469	45	232	146	836
vanilla ice milk soft serve	1 cup	223	5	38	13	163
vanilla ice milk soft serve	½ gal	1787	37	307	106	1303

ICES AND ICE POPS

FOOD	PORTION	CAL	FAT	CARB	CHOL	SOD
Ben & Jerry's						
Cherry Pop	1	330	24	28	55	—
Lemon Ice	4 oz	105	0	—	0	—
Raspberry	4 oz	105	0	—	0	—
Strawberry Ice	4 oz	77	0	—	0	—
Chiquita Fruit & Cream						
Banana	1 bar	80	2	—	—	—
Blueberry	1 bar	80	1	—	—	—
Peach	1 bar	80	1	—	—	—
Raspberry	1 bar	80	1	—	—	—
Strawberry	1 bar	80	1	—	—	—
Strawberry Banana	1 bar	80	2	—	—	—
Crystal Light						
Berry Blend	1 bar	13	0	2	0	2
Cherry	1 bar	13	0	2	0	4

FOOD	PORTION	CAL	FAT	CARB	CHOL	SOD
Fruit Punch	1 bar	14	0	2	0	2
Orange	1 bar	13	0	2	0	3
Pina Colada	1 bar	14	0	2	0	2
Pineapple	1 bar	14	0	2	0	2
Pink Lemonade	1 bar	14	0	2	0	2
Raspberry	1 bar	13	0	2	0	4
Strawberry	1 bar	13	0	2	0	2
Strawberry Daiquiri	1 bar	14	0	2	0	2
Dole Fresh Lites						
Cherry	1 bar	25	tr	6	0	10
Lemon	1 bar	25	tr	5	0	20
Pineapple Orange	1 bar	25	tr	6	0	33
Raspberry	1 bar	25	tr	6	0	5
Dole Fruit N' Cream Bar						
Peach	1 bar	90	1	18	5	15
Raspberry	1 bar	90	1	19	5	20
Strawberry	1 bar	90	1	18	5	20
Dole Fruit N' Juice Bar						
Pineapple	1 bar	70	tr	17	0	5
Pineapple/Orange/ Banana	1 bar	70	tr	17	0	10
Raspberry	1 bar	70	tr	15	0	15
Strawberry	1 bar	70	tr	15	0	10
Dole Sorbet						
Mandarin Orange	4 oz	110	tr	28	0	10
Peach	4 oz	110	tr	27	0	10
Pineapple	4 oz	110	tr	26	0	10
Raspberry	4 oz	110	tr	27	0	10
Strawberry	4 oz	100	tr	25	0	10
Dole SunTops, Grape	1 bar	40	tr	9	0	5

FOOD	PORTION	CAL	FAT	CARB	CHOL	SOD
Dole SunTops, Lemonade	1 bar	40	tr	9	0	5
Dole SunTops, Orange	1 bar	40	tr	9	0	5
Fi-Bar Juice Bar, Strawberry Nectar	1 bar	63	tr	15	—	—
Fi-Bar Juice Bar, Tropical Delight	1 bar	63	tr	15	—	—
Frusen Gladje Sorbet, Raspberry	½ cup	140	0	36	0	10
Good Humor Calippo, Lemon	4.5 oz	112	tr	—	—	—
Good Humor Calippo, Orange	4.5 oz	110	tr	—	—	—
Good Humor Ice Stripes, Cherry/Orange	1.5 oz	35	0	—	0	—
Good Humor Ice Stripes, Grape-Lemon	1.5 oz	35	0	—	0	—
Good Humor Italian Ice, Cherry	6 oz	138	tr	—	0	—
Good Humor Italian Ice, Orange/Raspberry	6 fl oz	138	tr	—	0	—
Good Humor Italian Ice, Watermelon	6 fl oz	138	tr	—	0	—
Good Humor Italian Ice, White Lemon	6 fl oz	138	tr	—	0	—
Haagen-Dazs Sorbet & Cream, Blueberry	4 oz	190	8	25	—	35
Haagen-Dazs Sorbet & Cream, Keylime	4 oz	190	7	29	—	30
Haagen-Dazs Sorbet & Cream, Orange	4 oz	190	8	27	—	35
Haagen-Dazs Sorbet & Cream, Raspberry	4 oz	180	8	23	—	35

FOOD	PORTION	CAL	FAT	CARB	CHOL	SOD
Ice, All Flavors (Bresler's)	3.5 oz	120	0	30	0	—
Jell-O						
Berry Punch	1 bar	31	tr	7	0	23
Lemon Lime	1 bar	33	tr	8	—	23
Mixed Berry	1 bar	31	tr	7	0	23
Orange	1 bar	31	tr	7	0	23
Orange Pineapple	1 bar	31	tr	7	0	23
Raspberry	1 bar	29	tr	7	0	24
Raspberry Peach	1 bar	29	tr	7	0	24
Side By Side Apple Cherry	1 bar	36	tr	8	—	7
Side by Side Grape Lemon	1 bar	36	tr	8	—	7
Strawberry	1 bar	31	tr	7	0	23
Strawberry Banana	1 bar	31	tr	7	0	23
Kool-Aid Cherry	1 bar	42	0	11	0	2
Kool-Aid Grape	1 bar	42	0	11	0	2
Kool-Aid Mountain Berry Punch	1 bar	42	0	11	0	2
Lifesavers Ice Pops	1	35	0	9	0	0
Lifesavers Ice Pops, Sugar Free	1	12	0	3	0	5
Vitari Passion Fruit	4 oz	80	0	—	0	—
Vitari Peach	4 oz	80	0	—	0	—

LIQUOR/LIQUEUR

FOOD	PORTION	CAL	FAT	CARB	CHOL	SOD
anisette	0.67 oz	74	0	7	0	—
apricot brandy	0.67 oz	64	0	6	0	—
benedictine	0.67 oz	69	0	7	0	—
bloody mary	5 oz	116	tr	5	0	332
bourbon & soda	4 oz	105	0	0	0	16

FOOD	PORTION	CAL	FAT	CARB	CHOL	SOD
coffee liqueur	1.5 oz	174	tr	24	0	4
coffee w/ cream liqueur	1.5 oz	154	7	10	—	43
creme de menthe	1.5 oz	186	tr	21	0	3
curacao liqueur	0.67 oz	54	0	6	0	—
daiquiri	2 oz	111	0	4	0	1
gin	1.5 oz	110	0	0	0	1
gin & tonic	7.5 oz	171	0	16	0	10
gin rickey	4 oz	150	0	—	0	—
manhattan	2 oz	128	0	2	0	2
martini	2.5 oz	156	0	tr	0	2
mint julep	10 oz	210	0	3	0	—
old-fashioned	2.5 oz	127	0	3	0	—
pina colada	4.5 oz	262	3	40	0	9
planter's punch	3.5 oz	175	0	—	0	—
rum	1.5 oz	97	0	0	0	0
screwdriver	7 oz	174	tr	18	0	2
sloe gin fizz	2.5 oz	132	0	4	0	1
tequila sunrise	5.5 oz	189	tr	15	0	7
tom collins	7.5 oz	121	0	3	0	39
vodka	1.5 oz	97	0	0	0	0
whiskey	1.5 oz	105	0	tr	0	0
whiskey sour	3 oz	123	tr	5	0	10
whiskey sour mix, as prep	3.6 oz	169	0	16	0	48
whiskey sour mix, not prep	1 pkg (0.6 oz)	64	0	16	0	46

MINERAL/BOTTLED WATER

FOOD	PORTION	CAL	FAT	CARB	CHOL	SOD
Artesia	7 oz	0	0	—	0	—
Artesia Almund	7 oz	0	0	—	0	—

FOOD	PORTION	CAL	FAT	CARB	CHOL	SOD
Artesia Cranberi	7 oz	0	0	—	0	—
Artesia Lemin	7 oz	0	0	—	0	—
Artesia Orange	7 oz	0	0	—	0	—
Crystal Geyser Sparkling Cola Berry	6 oz	0	0	0	0	30
Crystal Geyser Sparkling Lemon	6 oz	0	0	0	0	30
Crystal Geyser Sparkling Lime	6 oz	0	0	0	0	30
Crystal Geyser Sparkling Mineral	6 oz	0	0	0	0	30
Crystal Geyser Sparkling Natural Wild Cherry	6 oz	0	0	0	0	30
Crystal Geyser Sparkling Orange	6 oz	0	0	0	0	30
Diamond Spring	1 qt	0	0	—	0	—
Evian	1 liter (33.8 oz)	0	0	0	0	5
Glenpatrick Spring Pure Irish	8 oz	0	0	—	0	—
Mountain Valley	1 qt	0	0	—	0	—
San Pellegrino	1 liter	0	0	0	0	41
Saratoga Sparkling	8 oz	0	0	0	0	tr
Schweppes Vichy	6 oz	0	0	—	0	—

MUNCHIES

FOOD	PORTION	CAL	FAT	CARB	CHOL	SOD
Apple Chips (Weight Watchers)	0.75 oz	70	0	19	0	110
Bakem-ets	21 (1 oz)	160	10	2	25	850
Bakem-ets Hot 'N Spicy	21 (1 oz)	150	9	1	25	750
Bugles	1 oz	150	8	18	—	290

FOOD	PORTION	CAL	FAT	CARB	CHOL	SOD
Bugles, Nacho Cheese	1 oz	160	9	17	—	250
Bugles, Ranch	1 oz	150	9	16	—	290
Carrot Lites (Health Valley)	0.5 oz	75	4	9	0	5
Cheese Balls (Lance)	1 pkg (32 g)	190	13	16	5	420
Cheese Curls (Weight Watchers)	0.5 oz	70	2	10	0	45
Cheetos (Cheddar Valley)	26 (1 oz)	160	9	16	0	240
Cheetos Crunchy	26 (1 oz)	150	9	17	0	310
Cheetos Curls	15 (1 oz)	150	9	17	0	270
Cheetos Flamin' Hot	26 (1 oz)	150	9	16	0	240
Cheetos Light	38 (1 oz)	140	6	19	0	280
Cheetos Paws	16 (1 oz)	160	10	15	0	310
Cheetos Puffed Balls	38 (1 oz)	160	10	16	0	360
Cheetos Puffs	33 (1 oz)	160	9	16	0	330
Cheez Doodles, Crunchy	1 oz	160	10	16	—	230
Cheez Doodles, Puffed	1 oz	150	9	16	—	360
Cheez Waffies	1 oz	140	8	14	—	420
Chex Snack Mix, Barbeque	⅔ cup (1 oz)	130	5	18	0	480
Chex Snack Mix, Cool Sour Cream & Onion	⅔ cup (1 oz)	130	5	19	0	300
Chex Snack Mix, Golden Cheddar	⅔ cup (1 oz)	130	5	19	0	300
Chex Snack Mix, Traditional	⅔ cup (1 oz)	120	5	19	0	320
Combos Cheddar	1 pkg (1.7 oz)	250	13	28	5	520
Cheddar Cheese Cracker	1 oz	140	8	16	5	300

FOOD	PORTION	CAL	FAT	CARB	CHOL	SOD
Cheddar Cheese Pretzel	1 oz	130	5	18	0	310
Cheddar Cheese Pretzel	1 pkg (1.8 oz)	240	9	33	5	560
Chili Cheese w/ Corn Shell	1 oz	140	6	17	0	420
Chili Cheese w/ Corn Shell	1 pkg (1.7 oz)	230	11	29	5	710
Mustard Pretzel	1 oz	130	5	18	0	300
Mustard Pretzel	1 pkg (1.8 oz)	230	8	35	0	500
Nacho	1 pkg (1.8 oz)	230	8	34	0	580
Nacho Cheese Pretzel	1 oz	130	5	19	0	320
Nacho Cheese w/ Tortilla Shell	1 oz	140	6	17	0	380
Nacho Cheese w/ Tortilla Shell	1 pkg (1.7 oz)	230	11	30	0	640
Pepperoni & Cheese Pizza	1 oz	140	7	17	5	280
Pepperoni & Cheese Pizza	1 pkg (1.7 oz)	240	11	30	5	480
Pizzeria Pretzel	1 oz	130	5	19	0	290
Pizzeria Pretzel	1 pkg (1.8 oz)	230	8	35	0	520
Tortilla Ranch	1 bag (1.7 oz)	240	12	29	5	610
Tortilla Ranch	1 oz	140	7	17	5	350
Cornnuts, Barbecue	1 oz	120	4	22	0	270
Cornnuts, Nacho Cheese	1 oz	120	4	22	0	180
Cornnuts, Original	1 oz	120	4	22	0	170
Cornnuts, Picante	1 oz	120	4	22	0	260
Cornnuts, Ranch	1 oz	120	4	20	0	190
Crunchy Cheese Twists (Lance)	1 pkg (42 g)	260	16	25	0	290
Doo Dads	1 oz	130	6	17	0	360

FOOD	PORTION	CAL	FAT	CARB	CHOL	SOD
Eagle Cheese Crunch	1 oz	160	10	16	0	310
Easy Cheddar Nacho	1 oz	80	6	2	20	340
Easy Cheese, American	1 oz	80	6	2	20	340
Easy Cheese, Cheddar	1 oz	80	6	2	20	360
Easy Cheese, Cheese 'n Bacon	1 oz	80	6	2	20	340
Easy Cheese, Sharp Cheddar	1 oz	80	6	2	20	360
Frito Lay Toasted Corn Nuggets	1.38 oz	170	5	29	0	265
Funyums Onion Rings	11 (1 oz)	140	7	18	0	265
Gold-N-Chees	1 pkg (39 g)	180	9	23	5	410
Hain Carrot Chips	1 oz	150	9	16	—	160
Hain Carrot Chips, Barbecue	1 oz	140	8	16	—	160
Hain Carrot Chips, No Salt Added	1 oz	150	7	16	0	30
Health Valley Cheddar Lites	0.75 oz	40	2	4	tr	35
Health Valley Cheddar Lites w/ Green Onion	0.75 oz	40	2	4	0	35
Munchos	16 (1 oz)	160	10	15	0	230
Pork Skins (Lance)	1 pkg (14 g)	80	5	0	20	270
Pork Skins, BBQ (Lance)	1 pkg (14 g)	80	5	0	20	400
Ritz Snack Mix, Cheese (Nabisco)	1 oz	130	6	18	0	350
Ritz Snack Mix, Traditional (Nabisco)	1 oz	130	6	18	0	300
Snyder's Cheddar Cheese Twists	1 oz	150	8	17	0	200
Kruncheez	1 oz	160	10	15	0	170

FOOD	PORTION	CAL	FAT	CARB	CHOL	SOD
Onion Toasters	1 oz	150	8	17	0	280
Snack Mix	1 oz	130	5	18	0	300
Sopaipillas, Apple & Cinnamon	1 oz	150	8	18	0	15
Ultra Slim-Fast Lite N' Tasty Cheese Curls	1 oz	110	3	20	0	360
Wheat Snax (Estee)	1 oz	100	tr	22	0	15

PEANUT BUTTER

FOOD	PORTION	CAL	FAT	CARB	CHOL	SOD
Arrowhead Creamy	2 tbsp	190	16	6	0	tr
Arrowhead Crunchy	2 tbsp	190	16	6	0	tr
BAMA Creamy	2 tbsp	200	17	6	0	140
BAMA Crunchy	2 tbsp	200	17	6	0	115
BAMA Jelly & Peanut Butter	2 tbsp	150	7	20	0	75
Erewhon Chunky	2 tbsp (32 g)	190	14	7	0	75
Erewhon Chunky, Unsalted	2 tbsp (32 g)	190	14	7	0	10
Erewhon Creamy	2 tbsp (32 g)	190	14	7	0	75
Erewhon Creamy, Unsalted	2 tbsp (32 g)	190	14	7	0	10
Estee Chunky	1 tbsp	100	8	3	0	3
Estee Creamy	1 tbsp	100	8	3	0	3
Health Valley Chunky, No Salt	2 tbsp	170	14	6	0	2
Health Valley Creamy, No Salt	2 tbsp	170	14	6	0	2
Hollywood Creamy	1 tbsp	35	3	1	0	25
Hollywood Crunchy	1 tbsp	35	3	1	0	25
Hollywood Unsalted	1 tbsp	35	3	1	0	0
Home Brand	2 tbsp	210	17	—	0	—
Home Brand Natural, Lightly Salted	2 tbsp	210	17	—	0	—

FOOD	PORTION	CAL	FAT	CARB	CHOL	SOD
Home Brand Natural, Unsalted	2 tbsp	210	17	—	0	—
Home Brand No-Sugar Added	2 tbsp	180	16	—	0	—
Jif Creamy	2 tbsp	180	16	6	0	155
Jif Extra Crunchy	2 tbsp	180	16	6	0	130
Jif Simply Creamy	2 tbsp	180	16	5	0	65
Jif Simply Extra Crunchy	2 tbsp	180	16	5	0	50
Peter Pan Creamy	2 tbsp	190	16	6	0	150
Peter Pan Creamy, Salt Free	2 tbsp	190	17	5	0	0
Peter Pan Crunchy	2 tbsp	190	16	6	0	150
Peter Pan Crunchy, Salt Free	2 tbsp	190	17	5	0	0
Reese's Peanut Butter Flavored Chips	¼ cup (1.5 oz)	230	13	19	5	90
Skippy Creamy	1 cup (263 g)	1540	135	38	0	1240
Skippy Creamy, w/ 2 slices white bread	1 sandwich	340	19	33	0	430
Skippy Super Chunk	2 tbsp (32 g)	190	17	4	0	130
Skippy Super Chunk	1 cup (260 g)	1540	138	36	0	1120
Skippy Super Chunk, w/ 2 slices white bread	1 sandwich	340	19	32	0	410
Smucker's Goober Grape	2 tbsp	180	10	18	0	120
Smucker's Honey Sweetened	2 tbsp	200	16	7	0	155
Smucker's Natural	2 tbsp	200	16	6	0	125
Smucker's Natural No-Salt Added	2 tbsp	200	16	6	0	<10
Teddie Natural Peanut Butter w/ No Salt Added	2 tbsp	200	17	—	0	—

FOOD	PORTION	CAL	FAT	CARB	CHOL	SOD
chunky	1 cup	1520	129	56	0	1255
chunky	2 tbsp	188	16	7	0	156
chunky w/o salt	1 cup	1520	129	56	0	44
chunky w/o salt	2 tbsp	188	16	7	0	5
smooth	2 tbsp	188	16	7	0	153
smooth	1 cup	1517	128	53	0	1234
smooth w/o salt	2 tbsp	188	16	7	0	5
smooth w/o salt	1 cup	1517	129	53	0	44

PEANUTS

FOOD	PORTION	CAL	FAT	CARB	CHOL	SOD
Cocktail, Lightly Salted (Planters)	1 oz	170	14	5	0	80
Cocktail, Unsalted (Planters)	1 oz	170	14	5	0	0
Dry Roasted (Frito Lay)	1.2 oz	190	16	7	0	300
Dry Roasted (Guy's)	1 oz	170	14	3	0	310
Dry Roasted, Lightly Salted (Planters)	1 oz	160	15	5	0	110
Dry Roasted, Unsalted (Planters)	1 oz	170	15	5	0	250
Fresh Roast, Lightly Salted (Planters)	1 oz	160	14	5	0	120
Fresh Roast, Salted (Planters)	1 oz	170	14	5	0	110
Honey Roasted (Eagle)	1 oz	170	13	7	0	130
Honey Roasted (Little Debbie)	1 pkg (1.13 oz)	190	15	9	—	15
Honey Roasted (Planters)	1 oz	170	13	—	0	—
Honey Roasted (Weight Watchers)	0.7 oz	100	6	7	0	100

FOOD	PORTION	CAL	FAT	CARB	CHOL	SOD
Honey Roasted Cinnamon (Eagle)	1 oz	170	13	7	0	90
Honey Roasted, Dry Roasted (Planters)	1 oz	160	13	7	0	90
Honey Roasted Maple (Eagle)	1 oz	170	13	7	0	90
Honey Toasted (Lance)	1 pkg (39 g)	230	17	11	0	240
Low Salt (Eagle)	1 oz	170	15	5	0	90
Party Peanuts (Fisher)	1 oz	160	14	—	0	—
Peanuts (Beer Nuts)	1 oz	180	14	—	0	—
Peanuts (Planters)	1 bag (0.5 oz)	80	7	3	0	55
Roasted w/ Shell (Lance)	1 pkg (50 g)	190	15	8	0	0
Salted (Frito Lay)	1 oz	170	15	6	0	170
Salted (Lance)	1 pkg (32 g)	190	15	7	0	105
Salted (Little Debbie)	1 pkg (1.25 oz)	220	18	7	—	115
Salted Tube (Lance)	1 pkg (42 g)	240	20	9	0	120
Spanish (Planters)	1 oz	170	15	3	0	100
Spanish, Raw (Planters)	1 oz	160	14	5	0	5
Spanish, Salted (Guy's)	1 oz	170	14	3	0	170
Virginia Fancy (Eagle)	1 oz	90	8	3	0	65
cooked	½ cup	102	7	7	0	240
dry roasted	1 cup	855	73	31	0	1187
dry roasted	1 oz	164	14	6	0	228
oil roasted	1 cup	837	71	27	0	624
oil roasted	1 oz	163	14	5	0	121
oil roasted w/o salt	1 cup	837	71	27	0	9
oil roasted w/o salt	1 oz	163	14	5	0	2
Spanish oil roasted	1 oz	162	14	5	0	121

FOOD	PORTION	CAL	FAT	CARB	CHOL	SOD
Spanish oil roasted w/o salt	1 oz	162	14	5	0	2
unroasted	1 oz	159	14	5	0	5
valencia oil roasted	1 cup	848	74	23	0	1111
valencia oil roasted	1 oz	165	14	5	0	216
valencia oil roasted w/o salt	1 cup	848	74	23	0	9
valencia oil roasted w/o salt	1 oz	165	14	5	0	2
virginia oil roasted	1 cup	826	70	28	0	619
virginia oil roasted	1 oz	161	14	5	0	121

POPCORN

FOOD	PORTION	CAL	FAT	CARB	CHOL	SOD
Cape Cod	0.5 oz	80	5	6	0	150
Cape Cod Light	0.5 oz	60	3	8	0	95
Cheetos Cheddar Cheese	0.5 oz	80	6	6	0	160
Chesters	0.5 oz	70	3	9	0	200
Chesters Cheddar Cheese	0.5 oz	80	5	7	0	200
Chesters Microwave	3 cups	110	7	13	0	170
Chesters Microwave Butter Flavored	3 cups	120	7	13	0	180
Chesters Microwave Cheese Flavored	3 cups	110	8	11	0	230
Cracker Jack	1 oz	120	3	22		85
Eagle	0.5 oz	80	6	6	0	150
Jiffy Pop Bag, Butter	3 cups	90	5	11	0	140
Jiffy Pop Bag Lite	3 cups	70	3	11	0	110
Jiffy Pop Bag Regular	3 cups	100	6	11	0	140
Jiffy Pop Glazed Popcorn Clusters	1 oz	120	2	25	5	120

FOOD	PORTION	CAL	FAT	CARB	CHOL	SOD
Jiffy Pop Microwave Butter	4 cups	140	7	17	0	270
Jiffy Pop Microwave Regular	4 cups	140	7	17	0	270
Jiffy Pop Pan Butter	4 cups	130	6	16	0	270
Jiffy Pop Pan Regular	4 cups	130	6	16	0	270
Lance Cheese	1 pkg (25 g)	130	8	13	5	280
Lance Plain	1 pkg (25 g)	140	9	13	0	210
Lance White Cheddar Cheese	1 pkg (25 g)	140	9	12	5	170
Newman's Own	3.33 cups	80	1	16	0	0
Newman's Own Microwave						
Butter	3 cups	140	7	18	0	150
Light Butter	3 cups	90	3	18	0	100
Light Natural	3 cups	90	3	18	0	100
Natural	3 cups	140	7	18	0	150
Natural No Salt	3 cups	140	7	18	0	0
Orville Redenbacher's Gourmet						
Hot Air	3 cups	40	tr	10	0	0
Original	3 cups	80	4	10	0	0
White	3 cups	80	4	10	0	0
Orville Redenbacher's Microwave						
Gourmet	3 cups	100	6	11	0	200
Gourmet Butter	3 cups	100	6	11	0	240
Gourmet Butter Toffee	2.5 cups	210	12	26	tr	85
Gourmet Caramel	2.5 cups	240	14	29	tr	90
Gourmet Cheddar Cheese	3 cups	130	8	14	2	280
Gourmet Frozen	3 cups	100	6	11	0	200

FOOD	PORTION	CAL	FAT	CARB	CHOL	SOD
Gourmet Frozen Butter	3 cups	100	6	11	0	240
Gourmet Light	3 cups	70	3	8	0	115
Gourmet Light Butter	3 cups	70	3	8	0	110
Gourmet Salt Free	3 cups	100	6	11	0	0
Gourmet Salt Free Butter	3 cups	100	6	11	0	0
Gourmet Sour Cream 'n Onion	3 cups	160	12	12	0	270
Pillsbury						
Microwave Butter	3 cups	210	13	20	—	410
Microwave Original	3 cups	210	13	20	—	410
Microwave Salt Free	3 cups	170	7	23	—	0
Pop Secret						
Butter Flavor	3 cups	100	6	11	1	170
Butter Flavor Singles	6 cups	250	16	23	0	310
Natural Flavor	3 cups	100	6	11	0	170
Natural Flavor Salt Free	3 cups	100	6	11	0	<5
Pop Qwiz Butter Flavor	3 cups	100	6	11	0	170
Pop Qwiz Natural Flavor	3 cups	100	6	11	0	170
Pop Secret Light						
Butter Flavor	3 cups	70	3	12	0	115
Butter Flavor Singles	6 cups	140	6	23	0	190
Natural Flavor	3 cups	70	3	12	0	160
Natural Flavor Singles	6 cups	150	6	23	0	320
Smartfood Cheddar Cheese	0.5 oz	80	5	7	6	130

FOOD	PORTION	CAL	FAT	CARB	CHOL	SOD
Smartfood Light Butter	0.5 oz	70	3	9	8	105
Snyder's Butter	1 oz	140	9	13	0	140
Snyder's Cheese	1 oz	150	9	13	0	240
Snyder's Cheese Gourmet White	1 oz	150	9	13	0	240
Ultra Slim-Fast Lite N' Tasty	0.5 oz	60	2	10	0	150
Weight Watchers Microwave	1 oz	100	1	22	0	5
Ready-to-Eat Butter	0.7 oz	90	3	13	—	100
Ready-to-Eat White Cheddar Cheese	0.7 oz	90	4	11	—	120
Wise Tender Eating	0.5 oz	70	6	4	—	120
Wise w/ Real Premium White Cheddar Cheese	0.5 oz	70	5	4	—	170
air-popped	1 cup	30	tr	6	0	tr
popped w/ vegetable oil	1 cup	55	3	6	0	86
sugar-syrup coated	1 cup	135	1	30	0	tr

PRETZELS

FAST FACT
Pretzels are the oldest snack in the world. In A.D. 610 monks in southern France gave them to children as rewards for learning their prayers.

FOOD	PORTION	CAL	FAT	CARB	CHOL	SOD
A & Eagle	1 oz	110	2	22	0	570
A & Eagle Beer	1 oz	110	2	22	0	610
Estee Unsalted	7	50	tr	11	0	0
J&J Soft	1 (2.25 oz)	170	0	37	0	140
J&J Soft Bites	5	110	0	23	0	95

FOOD	PORTION	CAL	FAT	CARB	CHOL	SOD
Lance Twist	1 pkg (42 g)	150	1	30	0	700
Mister Salty						
Dutch	1 oz	110	1	22	0	440
Fat Free Sticks	1 oz	100	0	23	0	380
Fat Free Twists	1 oz	100	0	23	0	380
Mini	1 oz	110	1	21	0	450
Twists	1 oz	110	2	21	0	580
Very Thin Sticks	1 oz	110	1	22	0	600
Mr. Phipps						
Chips	8 (0.5 oz)	60	1	10	0	310
Fat Free Chips	8 (0.5 oz)	50	0	11	0	315
Lightly Salted Chips	8 (0.5 oz)	60	1	11	0	200
Sesame Chips	8	60	2	10	0	250
Quinlan						
Beers	1 oz	110	1	—	0	—
Butter Tiny Thins	1 oz	108	1	—	0	—
Cheese Tiny Thins	1 oz	109	2	—	0	—
Hard Sour Dough Thins	1 oz	100	0	—	0	—
Logs	1 oz	103	tr	—	0	—
Party Thins	1 oz	109	tr	—	0	—
Philly Style	1 oz	107	tr	—	0	—
Rods	1 oz	100	tr	—	0	—
Sour Cheese Tiny Thins	1 oz	100	0	—	0	—
Sticks	1 oz	105	tr	—	0	—
Thins	1 oz	104	tr	—	0	—
Tiny Thins	1 oz	109	2	—	0	—
Tiny Thins No-Salt	1 oz	115	2	—	0	—
Ultra Thins	1 oz	106	tr	—	0	—

FOOD	PORTION	CAL	FAT	CARB	CHOL	SOD
Rold Gold						
Bavarian	3 (1 oz)	120	2	22	0	430
Cheese Pretzel Chips	1 oz	120	3	22	0	240
Pretzel Chips	1 oz	110	1	22	0	310
Rods	3 (1 oz)	110	2	23	0	410
Snack Mix	½ cup (1 oz)	140	6	18	0	330
Sour Dough	1½ (1 oz)	110	2	22	0	230
Sticks	50 (1 oz)	110	2	23	0	490
Thin Twists	10 (1 oz)	110	1	23	0	510
Tiny Twists	15 (1 oz)	110	1	23	0	420
Seyfert's Butter Rods	1 oz	110	1	21	—	530
Snyder's						
Logs	1 oz	310	0	22	0	360
Minis	1 oz	310	0	22	0	460
Minis Unsalted	1 oz	310	0	22	0	70
Nibblers	1 oz	310	0	22	0	460
Old-Fashioned Hard	1 oz	100	0	23	0	590
Old-Fashioned Hard Unsalted	1 oz	100	0	23	0	80
Old Tyme	1 oz	310	0	22	0	310
Old Tyme Unsalted	1 oz	110	0	22	0	70
Rods	1 oz	310	0	22	0	320
Stix	1 oz	310	0	22	0	900
Very Thins	1 oz	310	0	22	0	570
Ultra Slim-Fast Lite N' Tasty	1 oz	100	tr	21	0	460
Wege Sourdough	1 oz	102	tr	23	0	548
Wege Unsalted	1 oz	102	tr	23	0	60
Wege Whole Wheat	1 oz	109	1	21	0	25
sticks	10	10	tr	2	tr	48

FOOD	PORTION	CAL	FAT	CARB	CHOL	SOD
thin twists	10 (2 oz)	240	2	48	0	966
twists	1 (0.5 oz)	65	1	13	tr	258

SHERBET

FOOD	PORTION	CAL	FAT	CARB	CHOL	SOD
All Flavors (Bresler's)	3.5 oz	140	2	30	6	—
Lime (Sealtest)	½ cup	130	1	28	5	30
Orange (Sealtest)	½ cup	130	1	28	5	30
Rainbow (Sealtest)	½ cup	130	1	28	5	30
Red Raspberry (Sealtest)	½ cup	130	1	28	5	30
orange	1 cup	270	4	59	14	88
orange	½ gal	2158	31	469	113	706
orange home recipe	½ cup	120	2	24	9	30

SODA

FAST FACT
On an average day, 965,000 Americans drink Coke for breakfast.

FOOD	PORTION	CAL	FAT	CARB	CHOL	SOD
Coca-Cola	6 oz	77	0	—	0	—
Coca-Cola, Caffeine-Free	6 oz	77	0	—	0	—
Coca-Cola, Cherry	6 oz	76	0	—	0	—
Coca-Cola Classic	6 oz	72	0	—	0	—
Coca-Cola, Diet Cherry	6 oz	tr	0	—	0	—
Crush Apple	6 oz	90	0	—	0	—
Crush Apple, Diet	6 oz	10	0	—	0	—
Crush Cherry	6 oz	100	0	—	0	—
Crush Grape	6 oz	100	0	—	0	—
Crush Orange	6 oz	100	0	—	0	—
Crush Orange, Diet	6 oz	12	0	—	0	—

FOOD	PORTION	CAL	FAT	CARB	CHOL	SOD
Crush Pineapple	6 oz	100	0	—	0	—
Crush Strawberry	6 oz	90	0	—	0	—
Crystal Geyser Mountain Spring Sparkler						
Black Cherry	6 oz	65	0	17	0	tr
Cranberry Raspberry	6 oz	65	0	17	0	tr
Kiwi Lemon	6 oz	65	0	17	0	tr
Peach	6 oz	65	0	17	0	tr
Vanilla Creme	6 oz	65	0	17	0	tr
Diet Coke	6 oz	tr	0	—	0	—
Diet Coke, Caffeine-Free	6 oz	tr	0	—	0	—
Dr Pepper	1 oz	13	0	—	0	—
Dr Pepper, Diet	1 oz	tr	0	—	0	—
Fanta Ginger Ale	6 oz	63	0	—	0	—
Fanta Grape	6 oz	86	0	—	0	—
Fanta Orange	6 oz	88	0	—	0	—
Fanta Root Beer	6 oz	78	0	—	0	—
Fresca	6 oz	2	0	—	0	—
Health Valley Ginger Ale	12 oz	153	1	35	0	30
Old-Fashioned Rootbeer	12 oz	120	1	26	0	12
Sarsaparilla Rootbeer	12 oz	153	1	35	0	27
Wild Berry	12 oz	142	1	33	0	27
Hires Root Beer	6 oz	90	0	—	0	—
Hires Root Beer, Sugar-Free	6 oz	2	0	—	0	—
Jolt	12 oz	17	0	—	0	—
Like Cola	1 oz	13	0	—	0	—

FOOD	PORTION	CAL	FAT	CARB	CHOL	SOD
Like Cola, Sugar Free	1 oz	tr	0	—	0	—
Lucozade	7 oz	136	0	36	0	—
Manischewitz Seltzer, No Salt Added	8 oz	0	0	0	0	9
Mello Yellow	6 oz	87	0	—	0	—
Minute Maid Lemon-Lime	6 oz	71	0	—	0	—
Minute Maid Lemon-Lime, Diet	6 oz	10	0	—	0	—
Minute Maid Orange	6 oz	87	0	—	0	—
Minute Maid Orange, Diet	6 oz	4	0	—	0	—
Mr. PIBB	6 oz	71	0	—	0	—
Orangina	6 oz	80	0	19	0	0
Pepper Free	1 oz	12	0	—	0	—
Pepper Free, Diet	1 oz	tr	0	—	0	—
Ramblin' Root Beer	6 oz	88	0	—	0	—
Royal Mistic						
Caribbean Fruit Punch	16 oz	230	0	57	0	5
Grape Strawberry	16 oz	230	0	57	0	5
Sparkling w/ Lime Kiwi	11.1 oz	112	0	28	0	38
Sparkling w/ Mandarin Orange Pineapple	11.1 oz	120	0	30	0	18
Sparkling w/ Mango Passion	11.1 oz	112	0	28	0	34
Sparkling w/ Raspberry Boysenberry	11.1 oz	112	0	28	0	24
Sparkling w/ Royal Peach	11.1 oz	112	0	28	0	30

FOOD	PORTION	CAL	FAT	CARB	CHOL	SOD
Royal Mystic *(cont.)*						
Sparkling w/ Wild Cherry	11.1 oz	112	0	28	0	28
Sparkling Diet w/ Lime Kiwi	11.1 oz	0	0	0	0	<90
Sparkling Diet w/ Raspberry Boysenberry	11.1 oz	0	0	0	0	<90
Sparkling Diet w/ Royal Peach	11.1 oz	0	0	0	0	<90
Sparkling Diet w/ Wild Cherry	11.1 oz	0	0	0	0	<90
Royal Mistic 'N Juice						
Black Cherry	12 oz	146	0	36	0	26
Peach Vanilla	12 oz	146	0	36	0	18
Tangerine Orange	12 oz	146	0	36	0	30
Tropical Supreme	12 oz	152	0	38	0	14
Wild Berry	12 oz	156	0	38	0	30
Schweppes						
Bitter Lemon	6 oz	78	0	—	0	—
Club	6 oz	0	0	—	0	—
Ginger Ale	6 oz	63	0	—	0	—
Ginger Ale, Diet	6 oz	tr	0	—	0	—
Ginger Beer	6 oz	68	0	—	0	—
Grape	6 oz	92	0	—	0	—
Grapefruit	6 oz	77	0	—	0	—
Lemon Lime	6 oz	71	0	—	0	—
Root Beer	6 oz	75	0	—	0	—
Seltzer	6 oz	0	0	—	0	—
Seltzer, Flavored	6 oz	0	0	—	0	—
Sparkling Orange	6 oz	86	0	—	0	—
Tonic Water	6 oz	64	0	—	0	—
Tonic Water, Diet	6 oz	tr	0	—	0	—

FOOD	PORTION	CAL	FAT	CARB	CHOL	SOD
7-Up	1 oz	12	0	—	0	—
7-Up, Cherry	1 oz	13	0	—	0	—
7-Up, Diet	1 oz	tr	0	—	0	—
7-Up, Diet Cherry	1 oz	tr	0	—	0	—
7-Up, Diet Gold	1 oz	tr	0	—	0	—
7-Up, Gold	1 oz	13	0	—	0	—
Shasta						
Birch Beer, Diet	12 oz	4	0	—	0	—
Black Cherry	12 oz	162	0	—	0	—
Cherry Cola	12 oz	140	0	—	0	—
Citrus Mist	12 oz	170	0	—	0	—
Club	12 oz	0	0	—	0	—
Cola	8 oz	98	0	—	0	—
Cola	12 oz	147	0	—	0	—
Cola, Diet	8 oz	0	0	—	0	—
Collins	12 oz	118	0	—	0	—
Creme	12 oz	154	0	—	0	—
Dr. Diablo	12 oz	140	0	—	0	—
Free Cola	12 oz	151	0	—	0	—
Fruit Punch	12 oz	173	0	—	0	—
Ginger Ale	8 oz	80	0	—	0	—
Ginger Ale	12 oz	120	0	—	0	—
Ginger Ale, Diet	8 oz	0	0	—	0	—
Grape	12 oz	177	0	—	0	—
Lemon Lime	8 oz	97	0	—	0	—
Lemon Lime	12 oz	146	0	—	0	—
Lemon Lime, Diet	8 oz	0	0	—	0	—
Orange	12 oz	177	0	—	0	—
Red Berry	12 oz	158	0	—	0	—
Red Pop	12 oz	158	0	—	0	—

FOOD	PORTION	CAL	FAT	CARB	CHOL	SOD
Shasta *(cont.)*						
Root Beer	12 oz	154	0	—	0	—
Strawberry	12 oz	4	0	—	0	—
Tonic Water	12 oz	0	0	—	0	—
Sprite	6 oz	71	0	—	0	—
Sprite, Diet	6 oz	2	0	—	0	—
Sun-Drop	6 oz	90	0	—	0	—
Sun-Drop, Diet	6 oz	4	0	—	0	—
TAB	6 oz	tr	0	—	0	—
TAB Caffeine-Free	6 oz	tr	0	—	0	—
Welch's Sparkling Apple	12 oz	180	0	—	0	—
Welch's Sparkling Grape	12 oz	180	0	—	0	—
Welch's Sparkling Orange	12 oz	180	0	—	0	—
Welch's Sparkling Strawberry	12 oz	180	0	—	0	—
Yoo-Hoo	9 oz	150	tr	31	0	200
club	12 oz	0	0	0	0	75
cola	12 oz	151	tr	39	0	14
cream	12 oz	191	0	49	0	43
diet cola	12 oz	2	0	tr	0	21
diet cola w/ Nutrasweet	12 oz	2	0	tr	0	21
diet cola w/ saccharin	12 oz	2	0	tr	0	57
ginger ale	12 oz	124	0	32	0	25
grape	12 oz	161	0	42	0	57
lemon-lime	12 oz	149	0	38	0	41
orange	12 oz	177	0	46	0	49
pepper-type	12 oz	151	tr	38	0	38

FOOD	PORTION	CAL	FAT	CARB	CHOL	SOD
quinine	12 oz	125	0	32	0	15
root beer	12 oz	152	0	39	0	49
tonic water	12 oz	125	0	32	0	15

YOGURT

FOOD	PORTION	CAL	FAT	CARB	CHOL	SOD
All Flavors (Cabot)	8 oz	220	3	42	10	120
All Flavors Ultimate 90 (Weight Watchers)	1 cup	90	0	13	5	120
All Flavors w/ Fruit Lowfat (Friendship)	8 oz	230	3	—	14	—
Amaretto Almond Yo Creme (Yoplait)	5 oz	240	10	—	30	—
Apple (La Yogurt)	6 oz	190	4	--	—	—
Apple Crisp Lowfat (New Country)	6 oz	150	2	30	—	85
Apple Original (Yoplait)	6 oz	190	3	32	10	110
Apples 'N Spice Nonfat Lite (Colombo)	8 oz	190	tr	38	5	140
B! Lowfat French Style (Colombo)	6 oz	140	3	22	—	105
Banana Custard Style (Yoplait)	6 oz	190	4	32	20	95
Banana Fruit On Bottom (Dannon)	8 oz	240	3	43	10	120
Banana Strawberry Classic (Colombo)	8 oz	250	6	42	—	140
Banana Strawberry Nonfat Lite (Colombo)	8 oz	190	tr	38	5	140
Banana Strawberry Nonfat Lite Swiss Style (Colombo)	4.4 oz	100	0	20	—	70
Bavarian Chocolate Yo Creme (Yoplait)	5 oz	270	11	—	30	—

FOOD	PORTION	CAL	FAT	CARB	CHOL	SOD
Black Cherry Classic (Colombo)	8 oz	230	6	36	—	140
Black Cherry Lowfat (Breyers)	8 oz	260	3	44	10	125
Black Cherry Lowfat (Light N' Lively)	8 oz	230	2	49	15	125
Black Cherry 100 Calorie w/ Aspartame (Light N' Lively)	8 oz	100	0	17	0	100
Black Cherry w/ Aspartame Cal 70 (Knudsen)	8 oz	70	0	12	5	75
Blueberry (Dannon)	8 oz	200	4	34	—	160
Blueberry (La Yogurt)	6 oz	190	4	—	—	—
Blueberry (La Yogurt 25)	8 oz	200	0	—	—	—
Blueberry (Mountain High)	1 cup	220	6	31	—	140
Blueberry Classic (Colombo)	8 oz	230	6	36	—	140
Blueberry Custard Style (Yoplait)	6 oz	190	4	32	20	95
Blueberry Fat Free (Yoplait)	6 oz	150	0	31	5	95
Blueberry Fruit On Bottom (Dannon)	8 oz	240	3	43	10	120
Blueberry Light (Yoplait)	6 oz	80	0	13	<5	80
Blueberry Lowfat (Breyers)	8 oz	250	2	48	10	120
Blueberry Lowfat (Light N' Lively)	8 oz	240	2	46	10	130
Blueberry Nonfat (Dannon)	6 oz	140	0	27	<5	105
Blueberry Nonfat Light (Dannon)	8 oz	100	0	17	<5	130

FOOD	PORTION	CAL	FAT	CARB	CHOL	SOD
Blueberry Nonfat Lite (Colombo)	8 oz	190	tr	38	5	140
Blueberry Nonfat Lite Swiss Style (Colombo)	4.4 oz	100	0	20	—	70
Blueberry 100 Calorie w/ Aspartame (Light N' Lively)	8 oz	90	0	15	0	110
Blueberry Original (Yoplait)	4 oz	120	2	21	5	75
Blueberry Supreme Lowfat (New Country)	6 oz	150	2	31	—	90
Blueberry w/ Aspartame Cal 70 (Knudsen)	8 oz	70	0	11	5	80
Blueberry w/ Aspartame Fat Free (Light N' Lively)	8 oz	50	0	8	0	60
Boysenberry Fruit On Bottom (Dannon)	8 oz	240	3	43	10	120
Boysenberry Lowfat (Knudsen)	8 oz	240	4	43	15	135
Boysenberry Original (Yoplait)	6 oz	190	3	32	10	110
Cherries Jubilee (Yoplait)	5 oz	220	8	—	30	
Cherry (La Yogurt)	6 oz	190	4	—	—	—
Cherry (La Yogurt 25)	8 oz	200	0	—	—	—
Cherry Custard Style (Yoplait)	6 oz	180	4	30	20	95
Cherry Fat Free (Yoplait)	6 oz	150	0	31	5	95
Cherry Fruit On Bottom (Dannon)	8 oz	240	3	43	10	120
Cherry Light (Yoplait)	4 oz	60	0	9	<5	75

FOOD	PORTION	CAL	FAT	CARB	CHOL	SOD
Cherry Lowfat (Knudsen)	8 oz	240	4	43	15	135
Cherry Lowfat (Light N' Lively)	4.4 oz	140	1	27	5	70
Cherry Nonfat Lite (Colombo)	8 oz	190	tr	38	5	140
Cherry Original (Yoplait)	6 oz	190	3	32	10	110
Cherry Supreme Lowfat (New Country)	6 oz	150	2	32	—	90
Cherry Vanilla (La Yogurt)	6 oz	190	4	—	—	—
Cherry Vanilla Lowfat Swiss Style (Lite Line)	1 cup	240	2	45	—	150
Cherry Vanilla Nonfat Light (Dannon)	8 oz	100	0	17	<5	130
Coffee Lowfat (Dannon)	8 oz	200	3	34	10	120
Coffee Lowfat (Friendship)	8 oz	210	3	—	14	—
Coffee Nonfat Lite (Colombo)	8 oz	190	tr	38	5	140
Dutch Apple Fruit On Bottom (Dannon)	8 oz	240	3	43	10	120
Exotic Fruit Fruit On Bottom (Dannon)	8 oz	240	3	43	10	120
French Vanilla Classic (Colombo)	8 oz	215	7	30	—	140
French Vanilla Lowfat (New Country)	6 oz	150	2	31	—	90
Fruit Cocktail Nonfat Lite (Colombo)	8 oz	190	tr	38	5	140
Fruit Crunch Lowfat (New Country)	6 oz	150	2	30	—	90

FOOD	PORTION	CAL	FAT	CARB	CHOL	SOD
Grape Lowfat (Light N' Lively)	4.4 oz	130	1	24	10	70
Hawaiian Salad Lowfat (New Country)	6 oz	150	2	31	—	90
Key Lime (La Yogurt)	6 oz	190	4	—	—	—
Lemon Custard Style (Yoplait)	6 oz	190	4	32	20	95
Lemon Lowfat (Dannon)	8 oz	200	3	34	10	120
Lemon Lowfat (Knudsen)	8 oz	240	4	43	15	135
Lemon Nonfat Lite (Colombo)	8 oz	190	tr	38	5	140
Lemon 100 Calorie w/ Aspartame (Light N' Lively)	8 oz	100	0	16	5	150
Lemon Original (Yoplait)	6 oz	190	3	32	10	110
Lemon Supreme Lowfat (New Country)	6 oz	150	2	31	—	90
Lemon w/ Aspartame Cal 70 (Knudsen)	8 oz	70	0	12	0	125
Lime Lowfat (Knudsen)	8 oz	240	4	43	15	135
Mixed Berries Fruit On Bottom (Dannon)	8 oz	240	3	43	10	120
Mixed Berries Lowfat (Dannon)	8 oz	240	3	43	—	120
Mixed Berries Lowfat (New Country)	6 oz	150	2	31	—	85
Mixed Berry (La Yogurt)	6 oz	190	4	—	—	—
Mixed Berry Custard Style (Yoplait)	6 oz	180	4	30	20	95
Mixed Berry Fat Free (Yoplait)	6 oz	150	0	31	5	95

FOOD	PORTION	CAL	FAT	CARB	CHOL	SOD
Mixed Berry Lowfat (Breyers)	8 oz	250	2	48	10	120
Mixed Berry Original (Yoplait)	6 oz	190	3	32	10	110
Orange Original (Yoplait)	6 oz	190	3	32	10	110
Orange Supreme Lowfat (New Country)	6 oz	150	2	31	—	90
Peach (La Yogurt)	6 oz	190	4	—	—	—
Peach Fat Free (Yoplait)	6 oz	150	0	31	5	95
Peach Fruit Mousette (Colombo)	3.5 oz	80	tr	14	<5	55
Peach Fruit On Bottom (Dannon)	8 oz	240	3	43	10	120
Peach Light (Yoplait)	4 oz	60	0	9	<5	75
Peach Lowfat (Breyers)	8 oz	250	2	48	10	120
Peach Lowfat (Knudsen)	8 oz	240	4	43	15	135
Peach Lowfat (Light N' Lively)	8 oz	240	2	46	15	120
Peach Lowfat Blended w/ Fruit (Dannon)	4.4 oz	130	2	24	5	80
Peach Melba Classic (Colombo)	8 oz	230	6	36	—	140
Peach Nonfat (Dannon)	6 oz	140	0	27	<5	105
Peach Nonfat Light (Dannon)	8 oz	100	0	17	<5	130
Peach Nonfat Lite (Colombo)	8 oz	190	tr	38	5	140
Peach Nonfat Lite Swiss Style (Colombo)	4.4 oz	100	0	20	—	70

FOOD	PORTION	CAL	FAT	CARB	CHOL	SOD
Peach 100 Calorie w/ Aspartame (Light N' Lively)	8 oz	100	0	16	5	115
Peach Original (Yoplait)	4 oz	120	2	21	5	75
Peach w/ Aspartame Cal 70 (Knudsen)	8 oz	70	0	11	0	95
Peaches 'n Cream Lowfat (New Country)	6 oz	150	2	31	—	90
Pina Colada (La Yogurt)	6 oz	190	4	—	—	—
Pina Colada Fruit On Bottom (Dannon)	8 oz	240	3	43	10	120
Pina Colada Original (Yoplait)	6 oz	190	3	32	10	110
Pineapple Lowfat (Breyers)	8 oz	250	2	47	10	120
Pineapple Lowfat (Light N' Lively)	8 oz	230	2	50	10	120
Pineapple Original (Yoplait)	6 oz	190	3	32	10	110
Pineapple w/ Aspartame Cal 70 (Knudsen)	8 oz	70	0	12	0	125
Plain (Cabot)	8 oz	140	4	16	14	160
Plain (Friendship)	8 oz	170	8	—	30	—
Plain (La Yogurt)	6 oz	140	6	—	—	—
Plain (Mountain High)	1 cup	200	9	16	—	140
Plain Classic (Colombo)	8 oz	150	7	13	25	160
Plain Extra Mild Sweetened (Colombo)	8 oz	200	7	30	25	140
Plain Lowfat (Breyers)	8 oz	140	3	16	20	170

FOOD	PORTION	CAL	FAT	CARB	CHOL	SOD
Plain Lowfat (Dannon)	8 oz	140	4	15	15	125
Plain Lowfat (Knudsen)	8 oz	160	5	17	25	180
Plain Lowfat (Meadow Gold)	1 cup	160	5	16	—	160
Plain Lowfat Swiss Style (Lite Line)	1 cup	140	2	16	—	150
Plain Nonfat (Colombo)	8 oz	110	tr	17	5	160
Plain Nonfat (Dannon)	8 oz	110	0	15	5	140
Plain Nonfat (Weight Watchers)	1 cup	90	0	13	5	135
Plain Nonfat (Yoplait)	8 oz	120	0	18	5	160
Plain Original (Yoplait)	6 oz	130	3	15	15	140
Raspberries & Cream (Yoplait)	5 oz	230	9	—	30	—
Raspberry (La Yogurt 25)	8 oz	200	0	—	—	—
Raspberry Classic (Colombo)	8 oz	230	6	36	—	140
Raspberry Custard Style (Yoplait)	6 oz	190	4	32	20	95
Raspberry Fat Free (Yoplait)	6 oz	150	0	31	5	95
Raspberry Fruit Mousette (Colombo)	3.5 oz	80	tr	14	<5	55
Raspberry Fruit On Bottom (Dannon)	8 oz	240	3	43	10	120
Raspberry Light (Yoplait)	4 oz	60	0	9	<5	75
Raspberry Lowfat (Knudsen)	8 oz	240	4	43	15	135

FOOD	PORTION	CAL	FAT	CARB	CHOL	SOD
Raspberry Lowfat Blended w/ Fruit (Dannon)	4.4 oz	130	2	24	5	80
Raspberry Nonfat (Dannon)	8 oz	200	4	34	—	160
Raspberry Nonfat Light (Dannon)	8 oz	100	0	17	<5	130
Raspberry Nonfat Lite (Colombo)	8 oz	190	tr	38	5	140
Raspberry Nonfat Lite Swiss Style (Colombo)	4.4 oz	100	0	20	—	70
Raspberry Original (Yoplait)	4 oz	120	2	21	5	75
Raspberry Sundae Style (Meadow Gold)	1 cup	250	4	42	—	160
Raspberry Supreme Lowfat (New Country)	6 oz	150	2	—	—	90
Red Raspberry Lowfat (Breyers)	8 oz	250	2	48	10	120
Red Raspberry Lowfat (Light N' Lively)	8 oz	230	2	43	10	130
Red Raspberry 100 Calorie w/ Aspartame (Light N' Lively)	8 oz	90	0	15	0	105
Red Raspberry w/ Aspartame Cal 70 (Knudsen)	8 oz	70	0	11	5	80
Red Raspberry w/ Aspartame Fat Free (Light N' Lively)	8 oz	50	0	8	0	60
Strawberries Romanoff (Yoplait)	5 oz	220	8	—	30	—
Strawberry (La Yogurt)	6 oz	190	4	—	—	—

FOOD	PORTION	CAL	FAT	CARB	CHOL	SOD
Strawberry (La Yogurt 25)	8 oz	200	0	—	—	—
Strawberry Banana (La Yogurt)	6 oz	190	4	—	—	—
Strawberry Banana (La Yogurt 25)	8 oz	200	0	—	—	—
Strawberry Banana Custard Style (Yoplait)	4 oz	130	3	21	15	60
Strawberry Banana Fat Free (Yoplait)	6 oz	150	0	31	5	95
Strawberry Banana Fruit On Bottom (Dannon)	4.4 oz	130	2	23	5	65
Strawberry Banana Light (Yoplait)	4 oz	60	0	9	<5	75
Strawberry Banana Lowfat (Breyers)	8 oz	250	2	50	10	120
Strawberry Banana Lowfat (Dannon)	8 oz	200	4	34	—	160
Strawberry Banana Lowfat (Knudsen)	8 oz	250	4	43	15	135
Strawberry Banana Lowfat (New Country)	6 oz	150	2	31	—	85
Strawberry Banana Lowfat Blended w/ Fruit (Dannon)	4.4 oz	130	2	24	5	80
Strawberry Banana Nonfat Light (Dannon)	8 oz	100	0	17	<5	130
Strawberry Banana 100 Calorie w/ Aspartame (Light N' Lively)	8 oz	90	0	15	0	100
Strawberry Banana Original (Yoplait)	6 oz	190	3	32	10	110

FOOD	PORTION	CAL	FAT	CARB	CHOL	SOD
Strawberry Banana w/ Aspartame Fat Free (Light N' Lively)	8 oz	50	0	8	0	60
Strawberry Banana w/ Aspartame Cal 70 (Knudsen)	8 oz	70	0	12	0	80
Strawberry Classic (Colombo)	8 oz	230	6	36	—	140
Strawberry Custard Style (Yoplait)	4 oz	130	3	21	15	60
Strawberry Fat Free (Yoplait)	6 oz	150	0	31	5	95
Strawberry Fruit Basket w/ Aspartame Cal 70 (Knudsen)	8 oz	70	0	11	5	90
Strawberry Fruit Cup (La Yogurt)	6 oz	190	4	—	—	—
Strawberry Fruit Cup Lowfat (Light N' Lively)	8 oz	240	2	47	15	120
Strawberry Fruit Cup Lowfat (New Country)	6 oz	150	2	30	—	85
Strawberry Fruit Cup Nonfat Light (Dannon)	8 oz	100	0	17	<5	130
Strawberry Fruit Cup w/ Aspartame Fat Free (Light N' Lively)	8 oz	50	0	8	0	55
Strawberry Fruit Mousette (Colombo)	3.5 oz	80	tr	14	<5	55
Strawberry Fruit On Bottom (Dannon)	8 oz	240	3	43	10	120
Strawberry Light (Yoplait)	4 oz	60	0	9	<5	75
Strawberry Lowfat (Breyers)	8 oz	250	2	48	10	120

FOOD	PORTION	CAL	FAT	CARB	CHOL	SOD
Strawberry Lowfat (Dannon)	8 oz	200	4	34	—	160
Strawberry Lowfat (Light N' Lively)	8 oz	240	2	45	15	130
Strawberry Lowfat (Knudsen)	8 oz	250	4	45	15	135
Strawberry Lowfat Blended w/ Fruit (Dannon)	4.4 oz	130	2	24	5	80
Strawberry Lowfat Swiss Style (Lite Line)	1 cup	240	2	46	—	150
Strawberry Nonfat (Dannon)	6 oz	140	0	27	<5	105
Strawberry Nonfat Light (Dannon)	8 oz	100	0	17	<5	130
Strawberry Nonfat Lite (Colombo)	8 oz	190	tr	38	5	140
Strawberry Nonfat Lite Swiss Style (Colombo)	4.4 oz	100	0	20	—	70
Strawberry 100 Calorie w/ Aspartame (Light N' Lively)	8 oz	90	0	15	5	105
Strawberry Original (Yoplait)	4 oz	120	2	21	5	75
Strawberry Rhubarb Original (Yoplait)	6 oz	190	3	32	10	110
Strawberry Supreme Lowfat (New Country)	6 oz	150	2	30	—	90
Strawberry w/ Aspartame Cal 70 (Knudsen)	8 oz	70	0	11	0	85
Strawberry w/ Aspartame Fat Free (Light N' Lively)	8 oz	50	0	8	0	60

FOOD	PORTION	CAL	FAT	CARB	CHOL	SOD
Tropical Orange (La Yogurt)	6 oz	190	4	—	—	—
Vanilla (La Yogurt)	6 oz	160	4	—	—	—
Vanilla Bean Lowfat (Breyers)	8 oz	230	3	41	20	150
Vanilla Custard Style (Yoplait)	4 oz	130	3	20	15	70
Vanilla Lowfat (Dannon)	8 oz	200	3	34	10	120
Vanilla Lowfat (Friendship)	8 oz	210	3	—	14	—
Vanilla Lowfat (Knudsen)	8 oz	240	4	43	15	135
Vanilla Nonfat (Yoplait)	8 oz	180	0	35	5	140
Vanilla Nonfat Lite (Colombo)	8 oz	160	tr	30	5	140
Vanilla Nonfat Light (Dannon)	8 oz	100	0	17	<5	130
Vanilla Nonfat Lite Swiss Style (Colombo)	4.4 oz	100	0	20	—	110
Vanilla Original (Yoplait)	6 oz	180	3	29	10	120
Vanilla w/ Aspartame Cal 70 (Knudsen)	8 oz	70	0	11	5	90
coffee lowfat	8 oz	194	3	31	11	149
fruit lowfat	4 oz	113	1	21	5	60
fruit lowfat	8 oz	225	3	42	10	121
plain	8 oz	139	7	11	29	105
plain lowfat	8 oz	144	4	16	14	159
plain nonfat	8 oz	127	tr	17	4	174
vanilla lowfat	8 oz	194	3	31	11	149

FOOD	PORTION	CAL	FAT	CARB	CHOL	SOD

YOGURT, FROZEN

FOOD	PORTION	CAL	FAT	CARB	CHOL	SOD
All Flavors Gourmet Yogurt (Bresler's)	5 oz	145	2	28	9	—
All Flavors Just 10	1 oz	10	0	3	0	14
All Flavors Lite (Bresler's)	5 oz	135	0	30	0	—
Apple Pie (Ben & Jerry's)	½ cup (4 oz)	140	3	28	10	55
Banana Strawberry (Ben & Jerry's)	½ cup	130	2	27	5	30
Banana Strawberry (Edy's)	3 oz	80	1	15	5	40
Black Cherry Free (Sealtest)	½ cup	110	0	24	0	50
Blueberry (Edy's)	3 oz	80	1	15	5	40
Blueberry (Elan)	4 oz	130	3	23	11	50
Blueberry Cheesecake (Ben & Jerry's)	½ cup	130	2	26	10	40
Blueberry Softy (Dannon)	4 oz	110	2	21	5	65
Butter Pecan Softy (Dannon)	4 oz	110	2	21	5	65
Cappuccino Softy (Dannon)	4 oz	110	2	21	5	65
Caramel Almond Praline (Elan)	4 oz	150	4	26	10	90
Cheesecake Softy (Dannon)	4 oz	110	2	21	5	65
Cherry (Edy's)	3 oz	80	1	15	5	40
Cherry Garcia (Ben & Jerry's)	½ cup	150	3	28	10	40
Chocolate (Ben & Jerry's)	1 pop (2.5 oz)	150	9	17	0	75
Chocolate (Ben & Jerry's)	½ cup	140	3	26	5	40

FOOD	PORTION	CAL	FAT	CARB	CHOL	SOD
Chocolate (Edy's)	3 oz	80	1	15	5	40
Chocolate (Elan)	4 oz	130	3	24	10	50
Chocolate (Haagen-Dazs)	3 oz	130	3	21	25	30
Chocolate Almond (Elan)	4 oz	160	6	22	10	50
Chocolate Bee-Lite	4 oz	100	tr	23	0	55
Chocolate Chip (Edy's)	3 oz	100	1	20	5	55
Chocolate Fi-Bar	1	190	7	26	0	160
Chocolate Free (Sealtest)	½ cup	110	0	24	0	55
Chocolate Fudge Brownie (Ben & Jerry's)	½ cup	170	4	31	10	95
Chocolate Kissed With Honey	3.5 oz	100	3	18	9	50
Chocolate Kissed With Honey Nonfat	3.5 oz	85	tr	19	0	60
Chocolate Nonfat Softy (Dannon)	4 oz	110	0	23	0	65
Chocolate Shake (Weight Watchers)	7.5 oz	220	1	44	5	140
Chocolate Softy (Dannon)	4 oz	140	2	25	5	65
Chocolate Yogurt Bar (Dole)	1	70	tr	13	—	50
Citrus Heights (Edy's)	3 oz	80	1	15	5	40
Coffee (Elan)	4 oz	130	3	22	11	60
Coffee, Decaffeinated (Elan)	4 oz	130	3	22	11	60
Coffee Almond Fudge (Ben & Jerry's)	½ cup	180	7	28	10	60
Cookies 'N' Cream (Edy's)	3 oz	100	1	20	5	55

FOOD	PORTION	CAL	FAT	CARB	CHOL	SOD
Dutch Chocolate Desserve	4 oz	80	0	18	0	62
Golden Vanilla Nonfat Softy (Dannon)	4 oz	100	0	22	0	65
Heath Bar Crunch (Ben & Jerry's)	½ cup	170	6	29	10	80
Lemon Meringue Softy (Dannon)	4 oz	110	2	21	5	65
Marble Fudge (Edy's)	3 oz	100	1	20	5	55
Peach (Elan)	4 oz	130	3	23	10	50
Peach (Haagen-Dazs)	3 oz	120	3	20	31	30
Peach Free (Sealtest)	½ cup	100	0	23	0	35
Peach Softy (Dannon)	4 oz	110	2	21	5	65
Peanut Butter Softy (Dannon)	4 oz	130	3	21	5	70
Perfectly Peach (Edy's)	3 oz	80	1	15	5	40
Pina Colada Softy (Dannon)	4 oz	110	2	21	5	65
Plain Softy (Dannon)	4 oz	90	1	17	5	60
Raspberry (Ben & Jerry's)	½ cup	120	2	24	5	35
Raspberry (Edy's)	3 oz	80	1	15	5	40
Raspberry Softy (Dannon)	4 oz	110	2	21	5	65
Raspberry Vanilla Swirl (Edy's)	3 oz	80	1	15	5	45
Red Raspberry Free (Sealtest)	½ cup	100	0	23	0	40
Red Raspberry Nonfat Softy (Dannon)	4 oz	100	0	22	0	60
Rum Raisin (Elan)	4 oz	135	3	25	12	55

FOOD	PORTION	CAL	FAT	CARB	CHOL	SOD
Rum Raisin Nonfat Softy (Dannon)	4 oz	100	0	22	0	65
Strawberry (Borden)	½ cup	100	2	19	—	50
Strawberry (Edy's)	3 oz	120	80	1	15	5
Strawberry (Elan)	4 oz	125	3	22	10	50
Strawberry (Haagen-Dazs)	3 oz	120	3	21	30	30
Strawberry (Meadow Gold)	½ cup	100	2	19	—	50
Strawberry Banana Softy (Dannon)	4 oz	110	2	21	5	65
Strawberry Banana Yogurt Bar (Dole)	1	60	tr	13	2	15
Strawberry Bar (Dole)	1	70	tr	15	2	25
Strawberry Fi-Bar	1	190	7	26	0	150
Strawberry Free (Sealtest)	½ cup	100	0	22	0	35
Strawberry Nonfat (Dannon)	6 oz	140	0	27	<5	105
Strawberry Nonfat Softy (Dannon)	4 oz	100	0	22	0	60
Strawberry Softy (Dannon)	4 oz	110	2	21	5	65
Vanilla (Edy's)	3 oz	80	1	15	5	50
Vanilla (Elan)	4 oz	130	3	22	11	60
Vanilla (Haagen-Dazs)	3 oz	130	3	20	40	40
Vanilla Almond Crunch (Haagen-Dazs)	3 oz	150	5	22	33	65
Vanilla Bee-Lite	4 oz	110	tr	23	0	55
Vanilla Desserve	4 oz	70	0	16	0	57
Vanilla Fi-Bar	1	190	7	26	0	150
Vanilla Free (Sealtest)	½ cup	100	0	23	0	45

FOOD	PORTION	CAL	FAT	CARB	CHOL	SOD
Vanilla Kissed With Honey	3.5 oz	100	3	17	9	75
Vanilla Kissed With Honey Nonfat	3.5 oz	85	tr	18	0	50
Vanilla Softy (Dannon)	4 oz	110	2	21	5	65

Do You Ever Eat in Any of These Restaurants or Chains?

Do you ever wonder exactly what you're getting in calories, fat, cholesterol, carbohydrates, and sodium?

Arby's, Au Bon Pain, Baskin-Robbins, Burger King, Carl's Jr., Church's Fried Chicken, Dairy Queen, D'Angelo's, Domino's Pizza, Dunkin' Donuts, Godfather's Pizza, Hardee's, Jack in the Box, Kentucky Fried Chicken, Long John Silver's, McDonald's, Pizza Hut, Ponderosa, Quincy's Family Steakhouse, Rax, Red Lobster, Roy Rogers, Shoney's, Taco Bell, TCBY, T.J. Cinnamon's, Wendy's, and White Castle . . .

These are just some of the establishments included in this comprehensive guide to fast-food nutrition.

ANNETTE B. NATOW, Ph.D., R.D., and JO-ANN HESLIN, M.A., R.D., are the authors of seventeen books on nutrition, including *The Antioxidant Vitamin Counter, The Cholesterol Counter, The Fat Counter, The Diabetes Carbohydrate and Calorie Counter, The Fat Attack Plan, The Iron Counter, The Pregnancy Nutrition Counter,* and *The Sodium Counter.* Both are former faculty members of Adelphi University and State University of New York, Downstate Medical Center. They are editors of the *Journal of Nutrition for the Elderly,* serve as editorial board members for the *Environmental Nutrition Newsletter,* and are frequent contributors to magazines and journals.

Books by Annette B. Natow and Jo-Ann Heslin

The Antioxidant Vitamin Counter
The Cholesterol Counter
The Diabetes Carbohydrate and Calorie Counter
The Fast-Food Nutrition Counter
The Fat Attack Plan
The Fat Counter
The Iron Counter
Megadoses
No-Nonsense Nutrition for Kids
The Pocket Encyclopedia of Nutrition
The Pregnancy Nutrition Center
The Sodium Counter

Published by POCKET BOOKS

For orders other than by individual consumers, Pocket Books grants a discount on the purchase of **10 or more** copies of single titles for special markets or premium use. For further details, please write to the Vice-President of Special Markets, Pocket Books, 1230 Avenue of the Americas, New York, NY 10020.

For information on how individual consumers can place orders, please write to Mail Order Department, Paramount Publishing, 200 Old Tappan Road, Old Tappan, NJ 07675.